YOUTHFUL

AGEING

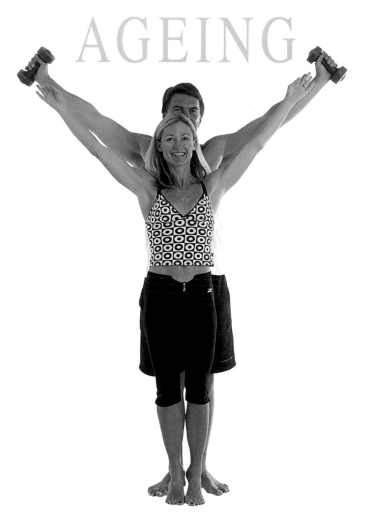

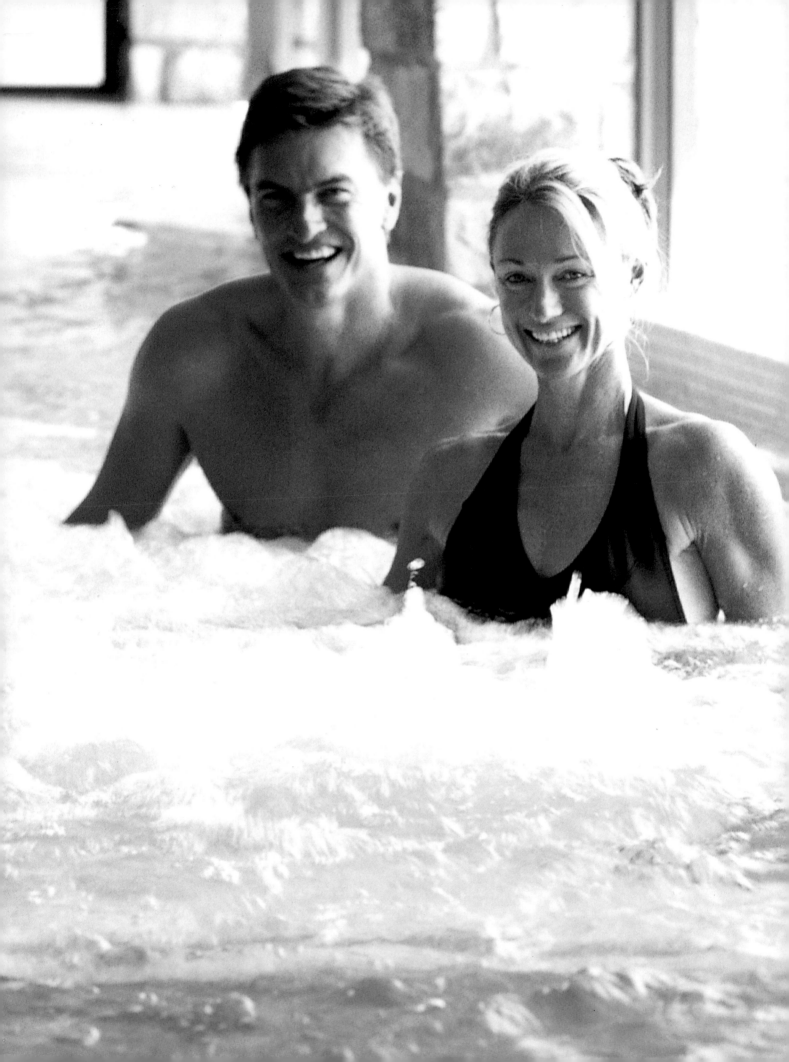

ANTI-AGEING
HANDBOOK

DR. GERALDINE MITTON

NEW HOLLAND

First published in 2004 by New Holland (Publishers) Ltd
London • Cape Town • Sydney • Auckland
www.newhollandpublishers.com

86 Edgware Road
London
W2 2EA
United Kingdom

80 McKenzie Street
Cape Town
8001
South Africa

14 Aquatic Drive
Frenchs Forest
NSW 2086
Australia

218 Lake Road
North Cote
Auckland
New Zealand

ISBN   (HB) 184 330 447 3
ISBN   (PB) 184 330 448 1

Publisher: Mariëlle Renssen
Publishing Managers: Claudia Dos Santos, Simon Pooley
Commissioning Editor: Alfred LeMaitre
Studio Manager: Richard MacArthur
Editor: Roxanne Reid
Designer: Lyndall du Toit
Illustrator: David du Plessis
Picture Researcher: Karla Kik
Production: Myrna Collins

Reproduction by Hirt & Carter, Cape Town, South Africa
Printed and bound in Singapore by Tien Wah Press (Pte) Ltd.

PICTURE CREDITS
AFP/PPCM p11 (bottom left). Corbis/Bettmann
pp111. Digital Source p118. galloimages/gettyim-
ages.com: pp10, 11 (bottom right), 15, 26 (top right),
29, 53 (bottom left), 58, 80, 84, 87 (bottom right), 100,
102, 105 (bottom right), 109, 113 (top), 120–21.
Gericke, Nick p26 (centre left). Hutchison Picture
Library: (Haslam, Nick) p75 (bottom right); (Murray,
Sarah) p12; (Woodhead, Leslie) p65 (bottom right).
imagingbody.com pp24, 35 (bottom right & left), 92
(bottom right & left); (Coates, Lionel) p84 (top right);
(Eurelios) p95. Mitton, Dr Geraldine pp25 (bottom
right), 103 (bottom left). Photo Access pp6, 22 (top
right), 41, 46 (top), 55, 57, 61, 63, 71, 93, 101, 113
(bottom right), 114; (Stephanie) p83; (Giraudon) p9.
Sycholt, August p47 (bottom left). Sylvia Cordaiy
Photo Library p112. The Image Bank pp27, 28, 45
(bottom left), 73, 108, 124, 125.

In memory of Cleto Saporetti,
philanthropist and visionary,
whose legacy will not be
forgotten.

Acknowledgments

I would like to thank Jill Singer for her help and encouragement, and for making my thoughts a reality, Alfred LeMaitre for guiding me through each chapter, and Roxanne Reid for organizing and editing my text with such clear understanding. Lyndall du Toit has made the book come to life with her inspired design and graphics, working hand in hand with photographer Warren Heath to portray the pathways to ageing youthfully.

Altira Wellness Spa, the Stellenbosch Hydro and Serenité Constantia Spa provided stunning settings for our spa and fitness therapy photographs and I am grateful for their generous assistance and co-operation. Thanks also to Dr. Nigel Gericke who has conducted research on the African herb Sutherlandia and has provided illustrations. Dr. Melodie de Jager, Brain Gym expert in South Africa, together with her publishers Human & Rousseau, kindly allowed us to use the Brain Gym exercises in Chapter Seven.

This book represents my own voyage of discovery, which started in a busy emergency department where I asked myself why relatively young people suffered heart attacks, strokes and lifestyle diseases, and why older people were so frail and dependent on multiple medications. I am grateful for my years with the Saporetti Foundation, which gave me the opportunity to travel internationally, as well as to research the effect of diet, natural therapies and mind-body interventions, and to practise what is now called integrative medicine.

Finally, I wish to express my love and gratitude to my sons Vincent and Mark, whose independence has allowed me the freedom to explore new paradigms of health.

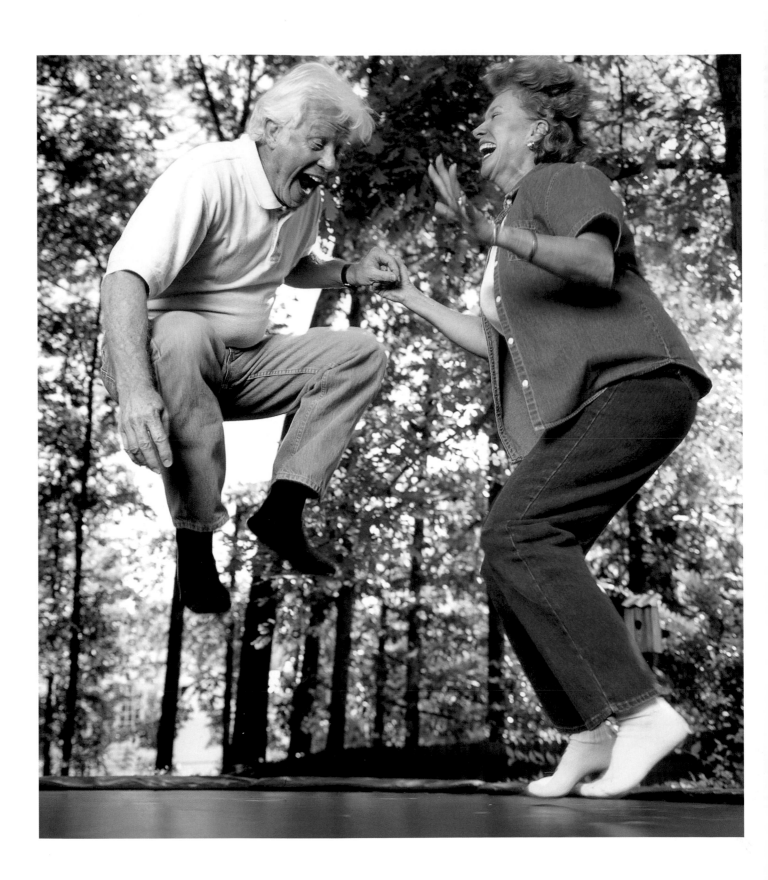

Contents

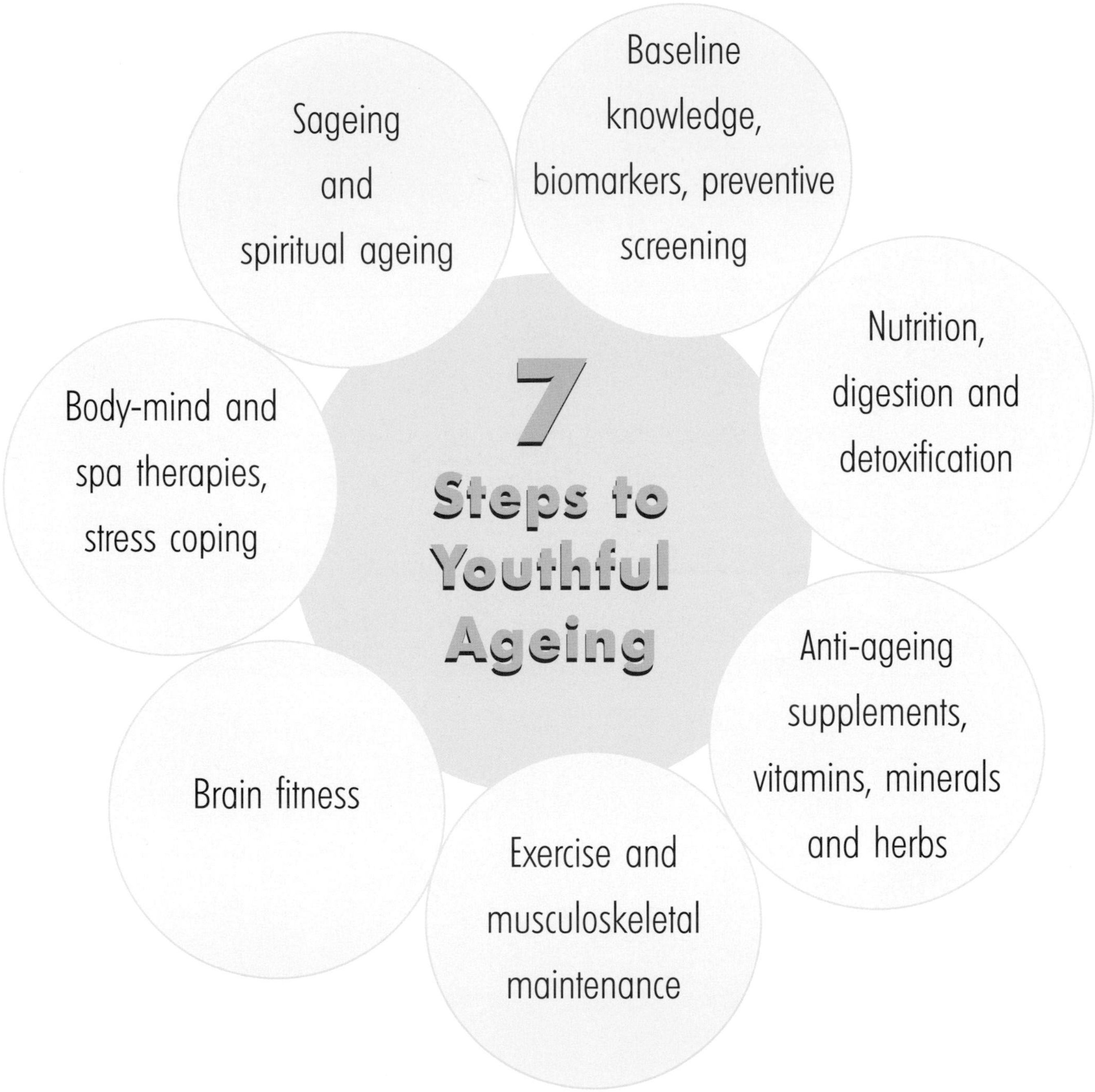

Sageing
and
spiritual ageing

Baseline
knowledge,
biomarkers, preventive
screening

Nutrition,
digestion and
detoxification

Body-mind and
spa therapies,
stress coping

7

Steps to
Youthful
Ageing

Anti-ageing
supplements,
vitamins, minerals
and herbs

Brain fitness

Exercise and
musculoskeletal
maintenance

WHAT IS YOUTHFUL AGEING?

'Every man desires to live long but no man would be old.' Jonathan Swift

Travelling back through the ages, there has always been a fascination with the process of ageing. Writers, scientists, doctors and explorers have searched for the 'fountain of youth'. Perhaps one day there will be a readily available and affordable magic bullet that will turn back the biological clock. This may be a fantasy today, but could it be a reality tomorrow?

In the past, we thought we were genetically programmed to age at a certain rate and in a similar way to that in which our parents aged. Our parents were old at 60, but what did they know about free radicals, insulin resistance, protein glycosylation and multihormone replacement therapy? We now know that only 10–15 per cent of our rate of ageing is inherited in our DNA. We are not programmed to die; we are programmed to survive. A mass of scientific research has shown that it is our lifestyle – what we eat, drink, breathe, think, believe, create and love – that determines our health and longevity. Age may be inevitable, but ageing is not.

One of the main features of the world's population in the 21st century has been a considerable increase in the number of older people in both developed and developing countries. This phenomenon is known as 'population ageing'. By 2020, the number of individuals aged 60 years and older will reach one billion. Currently, 20 per cent of the total Western world population is over 60, and by 2020 this will rise to 25 per cent. The 'oldest' country by 2020 will be Japan, followed by Italy, Greece and Switzerland. By 2020 the population of over-sixties in the United States will reach 23 per cent.

The rapidly growing number of older people means that more and more people will be entering the age when they are at risk of developing chronic degenerative diseases. In addition to the three leading causes of death – namely, cancer, heart disease and stroke – there is a growing number of people with mental health problems, Alzheimer's disease, Parkinsonism and age-related memory decline.

Today, we can expect to live to at least 78 years, up from 47 at the start of the 20th century. Medical advances will further increase life expectancy over the next two or three decades and we are told that it is possible for us to reach the age of 120.

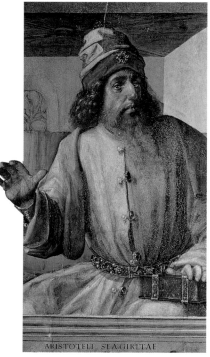

Aristotle

The notion of 'successful ageing' was probably first described by Aristotle, who used the term 'eugeria'. This he defined as living a long and happy life without suffering and without being a burden to others. In medical terminology we use the term 'progeria' to describe a syndrome of premature ageing.

The record in 1997 for the longest-lived person was the feisty Frenchwoman, Jeanne Calment, who celebrated her 122nd birthday before dying. Disproving the assumption that we will all develop Alzheimer's disease in old age, she displayed intelligence, humour and curiosity until the end of her days. There are many octogenarians today who are dancing, laughing, hoping, mingling, doing and helping their way to a youthful old age.

TOP 10 CHRONIC HEALTH PROBLEMS IN AGEING ADULTS

1. Arthritis
2. High blood pressure
3. Heart disease, circulatory disorders
4. Digestive problems
5. Diabetes, impaired blood sugar control
6. Bone and musculoskeletal problems, osteoporosis
7. Memory loss, Alzheimer's disease
8. Depression
9. Hearing loss, tinnitus
10. Visual impairment, cataracts, glaucoma, macular degeneration

MORE PROBLEMS FOR AGEING MEN

1. Prostatic hypertrophy
2. Hair loss
3. Gum disease
4. Declining hormone levels
5. Skin photo-ageing

MORE PROBLEMS FOR AGEING WOMEN

1. Underactive thyroid
2. Weight gain, metabolic syndrome
3. Urogenital ageing
4. Declining hormone levels
5. Skin thinning and wrinkles

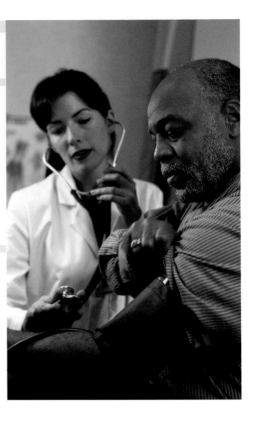

WHAT IS YOUTHFUL AGEING?

Good health and youthful ageing have many dimensions. This means having all your body parts in good working order; having a good memory, with precision in thought and action; having enough energy to enjoy physical activities; going to sleep and awakening easily; being able to laugh and be playful; being able to love and be loved, being able to enjoy the support of a wide circle of friends, being flexible and open to new adventures; being able to appreciate the beauties of nature and the environment; having a purpose and meaning to life; having spiritual well-being; and having 'joie de vivre'.

YOUR BODY AS YOU AGE

You are at your physical peak at the age of 35, after which it is downhill all the way – unless, of course, you choose to do something about it. The age of 40 is known as the chronological Rubicon, or 'the old age of youth and the youth of old age'.

One of the most noticeable changes after 35 or 40 is the change in body composition and the resulting change in shape. Muscle tissue is lost and replaced by fat. Muscle is metabolically more active than fat so you tend to gain weight as muscle or lean tissue is lost – especially around the middle. Lungs and heart become less efficient. Digestion may be compromised because gastric juices and enzymes decline, together with diminished absorption of nutrients.

The good news about brain cells is that although there is a little brain shrinkage, the connections between neurons can increase and be stimulated by mental and physical exercise. Bone density generally diminishes and the cartilage in the joints begins to deteriorate. Hearing may decline after the age of 65, teeth suffer from wear and tear, the superficial dermal skin layer becomes thinner and demonstrates photo-ageing. Waning hormones in men and women result in the andropause or the menopause, when many men develop enlargement of the prostate and both sexes may develop less efficient kidneys, with loss of bladder control.

If all this sounds depressing, there are definitely ways to combat and prevent age-related body decline, and it is never too late to start. This book will show you ways in which you can maintain and promote optimal health and function.

Throughout history there have been examples of individuals who have led long and productive lives. Michelangelo lived to the age of 91; Verdi composed operas in his seventies; Titian painted magnificent canvases when he was 80. These men lived at a time when the average life expectancy was less than 40. More recently, American artist Grandma Moses only started painting in her eighties. Apart from escaping life-threatening disease and infections, one wonders whether these people's ability to integrate right- and left-brain activities, together with an ongoing sense of purpose in their lives, was what helped to keep them healthy and well.

In years gone by, before the advent of antibiotics and good hygiene, it was infections such as pneumonia, tuberculosis and typhus that often led to an early death. Without techniques we have today, such as X-rays, blood tests, magnetic resonance imaging (MRI) scans, positron emission tomography (PET) scans, ultrasound and many other diagnostic modalities, early diagnosis of potentially treatable illnesses used to be impossible.

The recent ongoing New England Centenarian Study in the USA has identified certain characteristics of individuals who have reached the age of 100.
- They eat and drink in moderation.
- They stay in touch with friends and make new ones.
- They live in the present.
- They remain optimistic, with a positive attitude.
- They have a sense of humour, as well as a sense of mischievousness.
- They are interested in many things.
- They consciously challenge their brains.
- They have a purpose and are engaged in life.

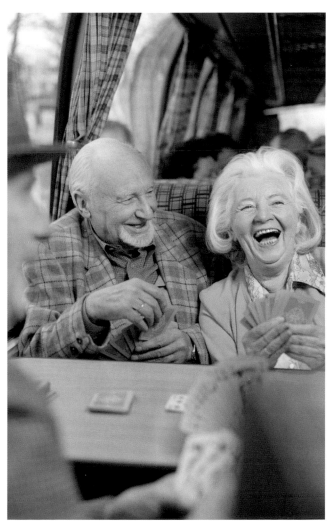

Enjoying companionship and new challenges, such as learning to play bridge, are vital for youthful ageing.

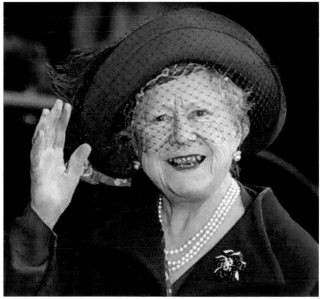

Britain's Queen Mum embodied many of the positive characteristics of centenarians, especially joie de vivre.

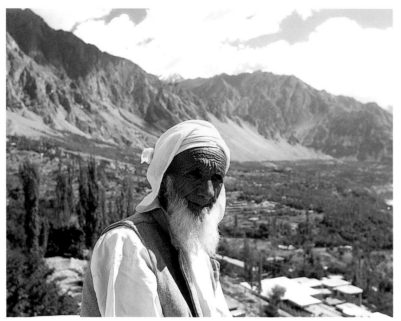

The secret of longevity of the Hunza villagers from the Karakoram Mountains of Pakistan is physical activity and a sparing diet.

There are communities where the population is known to be long-lived. What are their characteristics? The Hunza, who live an isolated existence in the Karakoram Mountains of Pakistan, eat sparingly of a largely plant-based diet uncontaminated by pesticides or artificial fertilizers. They drink unpolluted water, which has been washed down from glaciers and contains minerals. They are physically active and they fast when food is scarce.

The Italian community of Campodimele has been studied by the World Health Organization and found to have a life expectancy 20–30 years higher than the rest of Italy. Are the environmental influences in Campodimele especially significant? The village sits like an eagle's nest in the mountains south of Rome, accessible only by a narrow dirt road. Five generations of inhabitants work side by side in the fields, where they grow their own vegetables, especially tomatoes, cicerchia beans and fresh herbs. Their nutrition is simple and meagre. Corn is ground in a stone mill and baked in a wood oven. They consume home-grown olive oil and enjoy their own wine. They sing, eat joyfully and live in peace with themselves and with the environment.

The Okinawans live on a group of 160 islands between Japan and Taiwan. They have been the focus of an impressive 25-year study by researchers Dr Bradley Wilcox and Dr Makoto Suzuki. Average life expectancy in 2001 was 81 years – 86 years for women and 78 for men. With more than 400 centenarians in a population of 1.3 million, the statistics reveal 34 centenarians per 100,000 compared to 5–10 centenarians per 100,000 in the United States.

Do the Okinawans have the key to longevity? Research has identified certain characteristics that are common to most of them. Men and women of all ages have been shown to have a unique approach to healthy ageing that incorporates both Eastern and Western traditions.

• Their diet is based on plants, including tofu and seaweed. Importantly, they practise 'hara hachi bu'. This expression means that they eat until they are 80 per cent full, which helps to keep them slim and avoids obesity.
• Their daily exercise incorporates physical activity such as gardening, walking and martial arts.
• They practise the 'yin-yang principle', which stresses the need to achieve balance in daily living.
• They are spiritual people who have a deep and abiding respect for older people.
• They also practise a combination of Eastern and Western healing methods, some of which include the use of herbal remedies and psychospiritual practices such as meditation.

In the remote hills of southern China, known as the Bama province, live villagers in their eighties and nineties who are enjoying active and harmonious lives. The small population of 300,000 includes 80 centenarians – one of the highest ratios in the world. Although the media has focused on their enjoyment of rice wine and pickled snakes, their real secret is continued physical activity working in the fields, a frugal diet, an unpolluted environment, and the close family units of five generations all living under one roof. In fact, here we see a similar pattern to that of the Italians of Campodimele, the Hunza of Pakistan, and the Okinawans.

THE FUTURE OF ANTI-AGEING

For those who already have age-related or chronic degenerative disorders, there is hope on the horizon. Enormous strides have been made in the development of stem cells, tissue engineering and cloning. Embryonic stem cells are capable of developing into almost all cell types elsewhere in the body – for example, heart muscle, blood cells and neurons. They can thus act as a repair and replacement mechanism for a variety of damaged organs. Spinal cord injuries could be repaired by stem cells. Existing work with tissue engineering now also makes it possible to create new bone, new cartilage and new skin. Growing entirely new organs, such as livers, kidneys and hearts, will be a challenge for scientists in the future.

Telomere therapy is another emerging field of interest. Telomeres are the end segments of DNA on our chromosomes. Our body is made up of over a trillion cells. Each cell has 46 chromosomes and each chromosome has two ends, each with its own

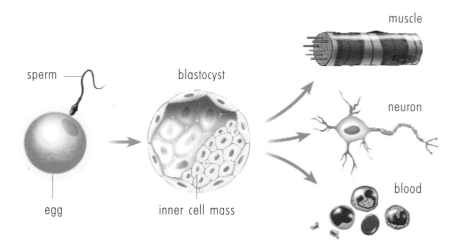

Stem cells can develop into muscle, brain or blood cells.

THE LONG AND THE SHORT OF TELOMERES

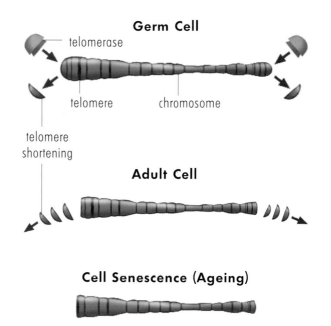

telomere, making a total of 92 telomeres per cell. Thus, in each individual there will be approximately ten quadrillion telomeres. Gradual shortening of these telomeres occurs over a period of time and results in cellular ageing. Can we treat chromosomes to lengthen telomeres in order to prevent further ageing or even to reverse ageing? Researchers are using the enzyme telomerase for this purpose.

We may be entering a new era in which doctors can extend human life, as well as prevent chronic degenerative diseases by repairing worn-out tissue. Dolly the Scottish sheep was cloned in 1997, and the cloning of human infants is in progress despite strong opposition. In the meantime, cloning of body parts is also underway, such as cloned teeth and hair. Perhaps male pattern baldness may even become a thing of the past before too long.

Anti-ageing medicine has become a fast-growing discipline and will be the medicine of the future, with the challenge of the 21st century being to prevent disease and disability. Although there are emerging frontier methods, the emphasis of this book will be on natural, healthy and optimal ageing rather than achieving life extension and longevity by technology and engineering. Its aim is to show that we need to concentrate on extending our healthspan rather than focusing on our lifespan.

Essentially, what we want is to live healthily, with a good quality of life, for as long as possible.

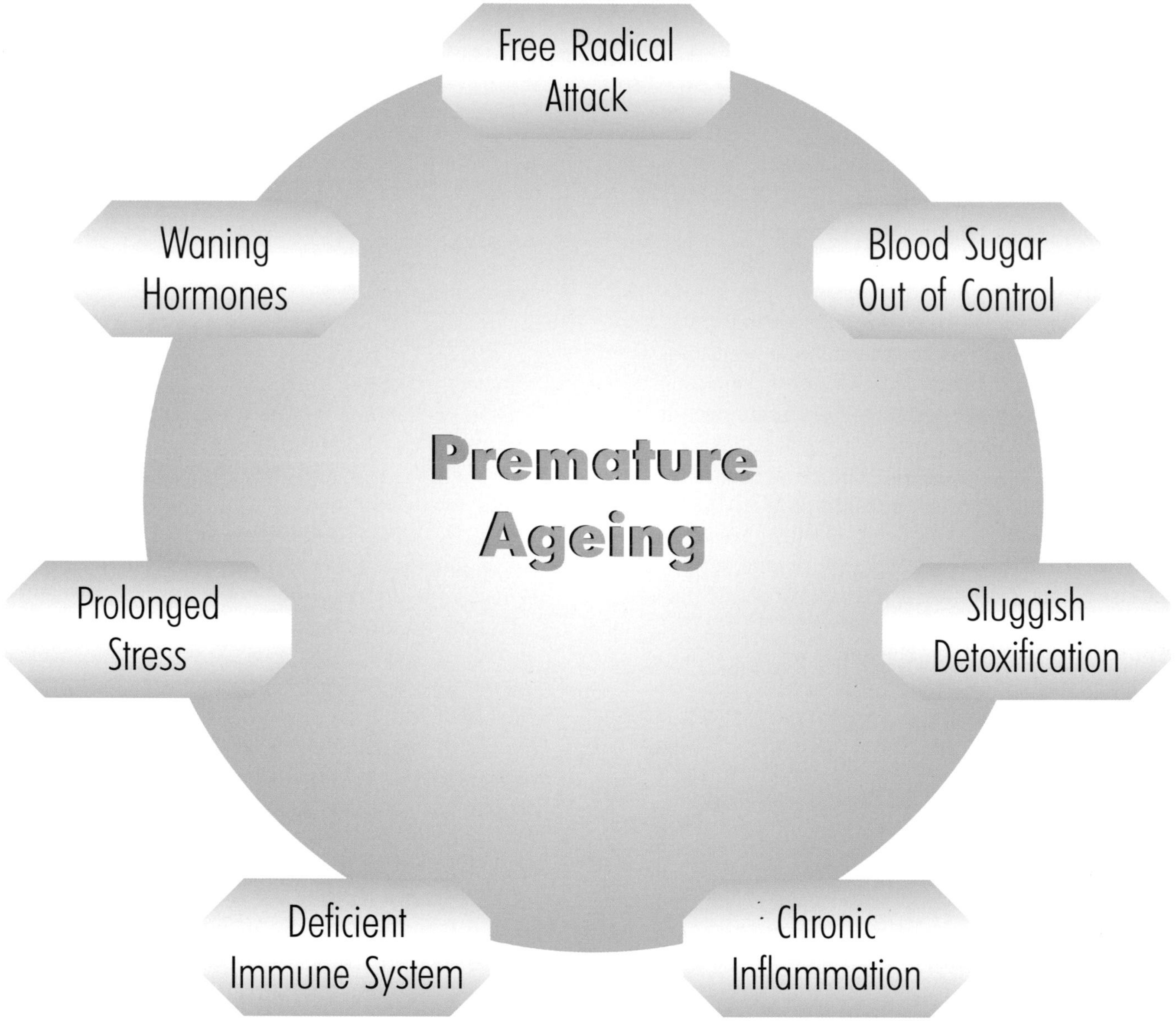

Free Radical
Attack

Waning
Hormones

Blood Sugar
Out of Control

**Premature
Ageing**

Prolonged
Stress

Sluggish
Detoxification

Deficient
Immune System

Chronic
Inflammation

ESTABLISH YOUR BASELINE KNOWLEDGE

Before you start taking steps to turn back the ageing clock, it is important to assess your current health status and establish baseline knowledge so that you can tackle any problems or defects. Abnormal function, as may be evident in laboratory tests, precedes disease. Screening and diagnostic tests may reveal potential future problems; you can then take preventive action to avoid disability or degenerative disease.

With the help of your doctor, you can undergo a number of tests to establish 'biomarkers' to monitor any age-related decline in your body's functions.

What is a biomarker? It is a means of measuring your rate of ageing by using physical and laboratory techniques. There are practitioners who measure chronological versus biological age based on questionnaires and lifestyle information. While these may be helpful, biological age cannot categorically be estimated from these. Your chronological age is the age that is registered on your birth certificate. Your biological age is the age you are estimated to be according to a number of parameters such as fitness, blood chemistry, cardiovascular health and general lifestyle factors. Some people look and feel much younger than their actual, chronological age, whereas others look and feel much older, irrespective of their response to questionnaires or computerized tests.

TESTS TO ESTABLISH BIOMARKERS

Depending on where you live, not all the tests mentioned will be available. Nutritional analysis and fitness testing are not essential, but blood pressure, blood sugar and urine testing *are* essential and there are always facilities for testing these, either at your doctor or your local pharmacy.

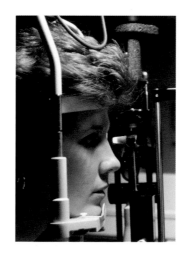

Eye test

At your doctor's or health practitioner's office
- Blood pressure and urine analysis
- Visual acuity, check for cataracts, glaucoma and macular degeneration
- Hearing test
- Skin examination, check for precancerous lesions
- Fitness testing, body fat analysis, body mass index (BMI)
- Nutrition analysis

Laboratory tests (blood, urine, saliva)
- Blood sugar profile, including fasting insulin and glycosylated haemoglobin (*see* page 21) to check on blood sugar control.
- Cardiovascular profile, including fasting lipogram, triglycerides, fibrinogen, homocysteine, and C-reactive protein (CRP).
- Basic blood profile, including electrolytes, kidney and liver function, thyroid function, complete blood count, and ferritin or iron levels. These are the usual tests that your doctor will prescribe annually.
- Age-related hormone profiles for men and women.
- Dehydroepiandrosterone (DHEA) is a steroid pre-hormone produced by the adrenal glands. The levels decline with age. DHEA may be prescribed as an anti-ageing supplement, so it is important to have your levels checked regularly. Adequate levels of DHEA may help to balance the negative effects of the stress hormone, cortisol, as well as contribute to overall wellbeing.
- The IGF-1 (insulin-like growth factor) test is a measurement of your growth hormone levels. A low level of IGF-1 suggests a low growth hormone level. Growth hormone declines with age, and until recently no intervention was considered necessary. If you

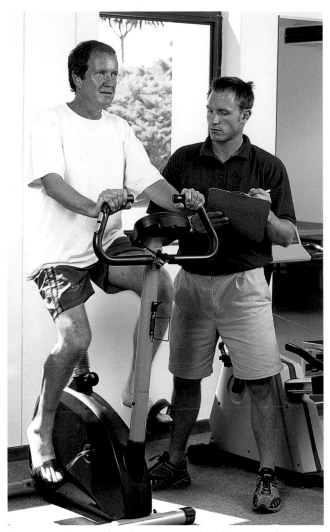

Fitness testing can be done at your local gym, and is individualized according to your age and health status. Aerobic fitness, muscular fitness and flexibility are important.

decide to take growth hormone (HGH), or perhaps even HGH secretagogues, which are amino acids stimulating natural release of your own growth hormone, the reason would be to restore some of the benefits of youth, especially a return to a youthful body composition. If you take HGH supplements, you must have IGF-1 levels checked every few months.

• Prostate specific antigen (PSA): this is a marker for prostate enlargement. Some 60 per cent of all men over the age of 50 develop prostatic hyper-

trophy or enlargement. As a high level of PSA may indicate prostate cancer, every man over 50 should have it checked annually.

• Immune cell subset: this blood test gives an indication of the health of your immune system. The immune system declines with age, so it is important to adopt measures that will keep immunity at peak levels.

• Vitamin and mineral profile, as well as an antioxidant screen, may be indicated if you have any symptoms of marginal nutrient deficiencies or if there are digestive problems, both of which are common with ageing.

• Free radical assessment (FRAS) may be done by a finger-prick or urine test, and is a useful indication of how many free radicals you are processing. If you live in an industrial or polluted area, are exposed to cigarette smoke, work with computers or take medications, this test will be a useful guide towards adequate antioxidant supplementation.

Mammogram and bone mineral density tests

Women are advised to have a mammogram at three-yearly intervals starting at 50 years of age. Ultrasound may be used in addition. Depending on individual risk factors, your doctor will advise you as to how often you should have a mammogram. Mammograms are not perfect as they miss about 10 per cent of all cancers. They involve a small amount of radiation, so their use remains controversial.

Screening for bone mineral density is recommended for women who have a family history of osteoporosis or other risk factors, such as smoking, steroid medications, eating disorders or excessive dieting, and for anyone who needs more information before deciding on whether to start hormone replacement or go the 'natural' route instead.

For both mammograms and bone densitometry, your doctor will refer you to a radiologist.

Now let us look at baseline tests for various age groups. These should be repeated annually or every two years, and will give an indication of your rate of ageing. The baseline tests in the table opposite provide a guide to tests that your health professional can arrange for you.

BASELINE TESTS FOR 40 TO 60 YEAR OLDS

IN YOUR FORTIES

· Blood pressure and urine analysis
· Body mass index, to estimate overweight or obesity
· Fitness testing, especially aerobic capacity
· Visual acuity
· Nutrition analysis
· Fasting blood sugar
· Cardiovascular profile
· Basic blood test profile
· Free radical assessment (FRAS)

For men:
· Cardiovascular risk factors

For women:
· Haemoglobin
· Ferritin levels
· Female hormone profile

IN YOUR FIFTIES

· Basic blood profile
· Blood pressure and urine analysis
· Skin examination
· Body mass index (BMI)
· Fitness testing, including muscular strength, flexibility
  and balance
· Visual acuity
· Blood sugar profile
· Cardiovascular profile, including electrocardiograph and lung
  function
· Free radical assessment (FRAS)

For men:
· Male hormone profile
· DHEA levels
· Prostate specific antigen (PSA)
· Digital rectal examination
· Colonoscopy, if risk factors are present

For women:
· Female hormone profile
· Thyroid hormone profile
· DHEA levels
· Mammogram
· Pelvic ultrasound
· Bone mineral density

IN YOUR SIXTIES AND BEYOND

· Blood pressure and urine analysis
· Skin examination, check precancerous lesions
· Visual acuity, check for cataract, macular degeneration, glaucoma
· Hearing test
· Basic blood profile
· Cancer markers
· Blood sugar
· Memory testing, cognitive function and reaction time

For men:
· Prostate specific antigen (PSA)
· Digital rectal examination
· DHEA
· Male hormone profile

For women:
· Bone mineral density
· Thyroid hormone
· DHEA
· Ferritin levels, check iron stores

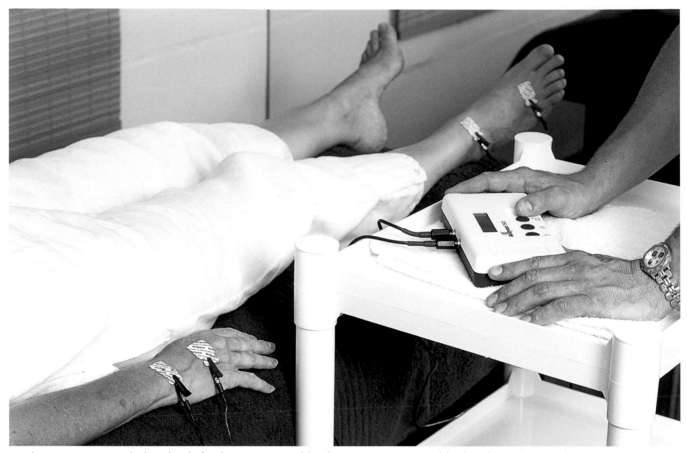

Body composition, including body fat, lean tissue and body water, is measured by bioelectrical impedance apparatus.

Measuring body composition

If you do not have access to equipment to measure body composition and body fat, such as bioelectrical impedance or skin calipers, there are two alternative methods for measuring overweight: body mass index (BMI) or waist circumference.

BMI does not take into account weight associated with fat and weight associated with muscle, so body build and proportion are not taken into account. Although a body builder may have the same BMI as an overweight man, it is still a useful tool for home use. BMI is an index of weight in kilograms, divided by height in metres squared. (To convert pounds to kilograms, divide by 2.2; to convert inches to metres, multiply by 0.0254.)

$$BMI = \frac{WEIGHT\ IN\ KG}{SQUARE\ OF\ HEIGHT\ IN\ METRES}$$

CLASSIFICATION	BMI	RISK OF ILLNESS
Underweight	< 18.5	Low
Normal range	18.5–25	Average
Overweight	> 25	Increased
Pre-obese	25–30	Increased
Obese	30–40	Much increased

Waist circumference is measured at the midpoint between the top of your hip bone (iliac crest) and the lower border of the rib cage. This gives an indication of the amount of intra-abdominal fat and therefore indicates your risk of developing Syndrome X or metabolic syndrome (*see* page 21), high blood pressure, heart disease, and diabetes.

In men: there is increased risk of these complications if waist measurement is more than 94cm (37in).

In women: there is increased risk of complications if waist measurement is more than 82cm (32in).

These measurements apply to Western European populations, and would differ according to different population groups.

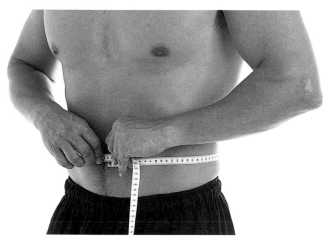

Measure waist circumference to show if you are overweight.

Thyroid self-test

The blood test for thyroid function is not always sensitive if there is marginal underactivity of the thyroid, known as subclinical hypothyroidism. Here is a test you can perform at home.

1. Take your underarm temperature first thing in the morning before you get out of bed. Keep still and quiet, and leave the thermometer in place for 10 minutes.
2. Take underarm temperature on five consecutive days. Keep a log.
3. If your temperature is consistently below 36.5°C (97.6°F), you may have an underactive thyroid. Consult your doctor.

SELF-EVALUATION QUESTIONNAIRE

· Do you eat less than five fruits and vegetables daily?
· Do you drink more than four cups of tea or coffee daily?
· Do you eat desserts more than twice a week?
· Do you snack on chips, biscuits, sweets or pastries?
· Do you consume more than two alcoholic drinks daily?
· Do you take prescription medications, such as sleeping pills, blood pressure pills, pain pills or anti-inflammatories?
· Do you regularly sunbathe, use tanning beds, play outdoor sport, or enjoy gardening?
· Do you smoke?
· Do you work in an industrial area, or is your home close to a busy road?
· Do you often suffer from colds and flu, or take antibiotics more than once a year?
· Do you suffer from indigestion, bloating or constipation?
· Do you have a family history of heart disease, diabetes or cancer?
· Do you suffer from insomnia?
· Do you find it difficult to relax?
· Do you often feel tense, irritable or angry?
· Do you suffer from headaches?
· Do you live alone?
· Do you have few close friends or family to act as a support system?
· Do you tend to be pessimistic rather than optimistic?
· Are you a couch potato?
· Are you constantly trying to lose weight?
· Is your memory not as good as it was when you were 30?

Each YES answer to these questions is a marker for premature ageing. As you read further in this book you will understand why these factors are ageing, and discover ways to halt the ageing process. For instance, there is no need for you to suffer memory loss as you get older.

SEVEN RISK FACTORS FOR AGEING

1. **Free radical attack**

2. **Out-of-control blood sugar**

3. **Sluggish detoxification**

4. **Chronic inflammation**

5. **A declining immune system**

6. **Prolonged stress**

7. **Waning hormones**

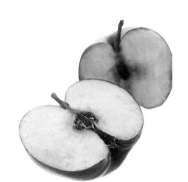

For you to understand the rationale for your baseline tests, we need to look at the risk factors for premature ageing.

1 Free radical attack

When an apple is cut in half, it turns brown as a result of a process known as oxidation. Our bodies undergo a similar process – akin to rusting – as a result of oxidation by villains known as 'free radicals'. Free radicals are highly reactive compounds produced during our normal daily metabolic processes. They are a major cause of ageing. Free-radical tissue damage results in coronary heart disease, brain damage, cancer and many chronic degenerative dis-

FORMATION OF FREE RADICALS

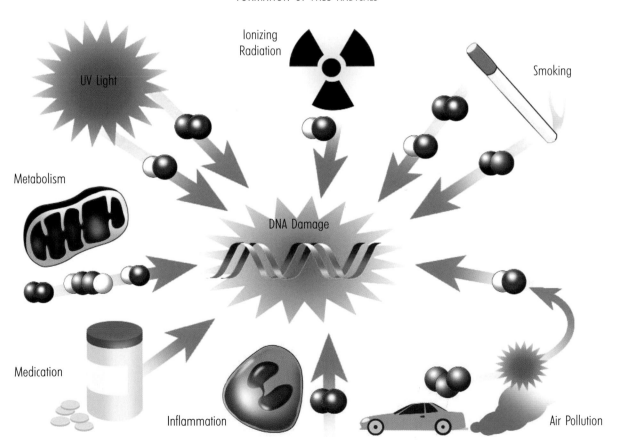

Our bodies are subjected to thousands of free-radical attacks every day.

orders. Free radicals are increased by cigarette smoke, environmental pollution, ultraviolet light, ionizing radiation, strenuous exercise and certain prescription medications. Free radicals damage cell membranes, paving the way, for example, for the onset of arthritis. They can also damage enzymes and genetic material of cells, leading to cancer. The body has a multilevel defence system to fight free radicals. This includes various enzymes that rely on the synergistic activity of antioxidant vitamins and minerals to activate them.

How can you combat free radicals?

To ensure that you have an army of antioxidant warriors, you need to consume a variety of dietary antioxidants, as well as supplementing – especially when you may be experiencing an excessive load of free radicals. Considering the stresses and environmental exposures of modern-day living, youthful agers would in general benefit from antioxidant supplementation.

The FRAS blood test is a test for free radicals. It is also possible to test for antioxidant status.

2 Out-of-control blood sugar

This is another factor causing premature ageing. Taken to extremes, excessive amounts of circulating blood sugar, together with inadequate insulin response, can lead to diabetes. Before this happens, a person may develop Syndrome X or insulin resistance, also known as metabolic syndrome. When glucose enters the bloodstream, the pancreas secretes insulin to deal with it, but if the cells become resistant to insulin, blood sugar goes out of control and insulin levels rise. Syndrome X is asso-

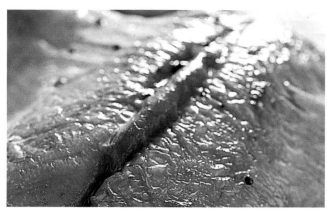

Glycosylation turns the skin of a roasted chicken brown.

ciated with abdominal obesity (apple-shaped obesity), high blood pressure and increased risk of heart disease. Other symptoms include mood swings, irritability, sugar cravings, episodes of hunger, and fluctuating levels of energy.

If you consume excessive amounts of sugar or refined carbohydrates in the diet, the result is a process known as 'AGE-ing'. Scientists have found that there is a process called glycosylation in which glucose combines with proteins in the blood or tissues, forming a sticky compound known as Advanced Glycosylated End products, or AGEs. A similar process can be demonstrated when a chicken is roasted: the browning of the chicken skin is a result of glycosylation. In the human body, AGE-ing results in tissue damage, auto-immune disease and chronic degenerative disorders.

The blood test for long-term blood sugar control is called glycosylated haemoglobin (HBA1C) and is part of your baseline blood sugar profile tests.

SYNDROME X = INSULIN RESISTANCE

When we eat carbohydrate foods, the body produces insulin to help carry glucose out of the bloodstream.

RESULTS:
1. Reduced ability to keep the blood sugar even
2. Cravings for sugar and carbohydrates
3. Central obesity
4. Adult onset of diabetes
5. High blood pressure
6. Increased blood lipids
7. Increased uric acid

How can you minimize blood sugar fluctuations?

1. Reduce the amount of refined carbohydrates in your diet, avoiding white bread, cakes, biscuits, sweets, cookies, desserts and sugar. Try to consume adequate amounts of protein and good fats. Being overweight is the main cause of Syndrome X, so weight loss is crucial. A high-protein, low-carbohydrate, normal-fat diet has been shown to be effective for weight loss but according to current research should not be continued for longer than six months. The large amounts of protein may have a negative effect on the kidneys and on bone density if continued indefinitely.

2. On the topic of weight control, remember that your metabolic rate slows down after the age of 40, so it is easier to gain weight while consuming the same number of calories. It is known that calorie restriction increases longevity, so you should eat smaller, nutrient-dense meals as you get older. You should also practise 'hara hachi bu' like the Okinawans (*see* page 12), who eat until they are 80 per cent full.

3. Alpha lipoic acid (ALA) and carnosine both protect against AGE-ing or protein glycosylation, and would be beneficial in the treatment of blood sugar disorders.

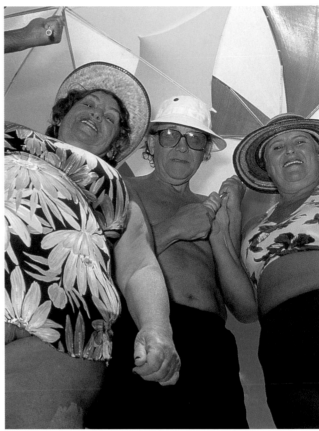

Abdominal fat is often associated with blood sugar problems, high blood pressure, increased risk of heart disease and onset of adult diabetes.

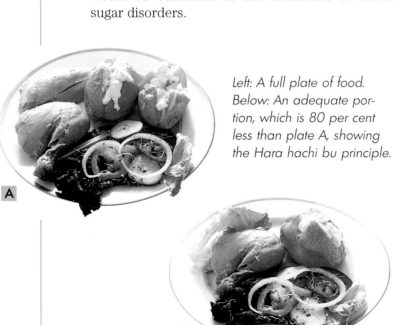

Left: A full plate of food. Below: An adequate portion, which is 80 per cent less than plate A, showing the Hara hachi bu principle.

A

B

3 Sluggish detoxification

During our lifetime we consume at least 25 tons of food. It is quite remarkable to think that due to the efficiency of our digestive tract and liver this amount of food is processed, digested and assimilated. This aspect will be discussed further in the next chapter (*see* pages 35–37).

Toxins found in your drinking water, environment, food, and especially in medications, create a serious load on the detoxification processes of your liver. An unhealthy intestine also produces an ongoing source of toxins.

Impaired detoxification is one of the most serious causes of premature ageing. Conversely, avoidance of toxins is one of the most effective ways to maintain and improve your health.

What are the signs of impaired detoxification?
- A feeling of 'hangover' even without alcohol
- Chonic tiredness
- Bad breath
- Migraines
- Chemical sensitivity, e.g. sulphites in commercial salads, wine and dried fruits
- Itching skin, nose and ears
- Skin allergies, urticaria and eczema
- Caffeine intolerance (small amounts keep you awake at night even if consumed early in the day)
- Joint pains and stiffness
- Irritable bowel syndrome
- Premature development of skin pigmentation, 'liver' or age spots

How can you decrease your toxic load?
- Avoid additives and preservatives, packaged and processed foods.
- Eat an abundance of raw or lightly steamed organic vegetables.
- Limit alcohol intake to less than two drinks daily.
- Drink six to eight glasses of filtered water a day.
- Restrict your use of anti-inflammatory drugs and antibiotics.
- Eat probiotic foods (e.g. yoghurt) and fermented foods (e.g. sauerkraut) to encourage a healthy gut.
- Eat prebiotic foods, such as banana and asparagus, which act synergistically with probiotics.
- Eat plenty of fibre, garlic and beetroot.
- Do a modified fast (*see* page 36) one day a week and a seven-day detox programme (*see* page 37) every three to four months.

Detoxification will be discussed in detail in the next chapter (*see* pages 35–37).

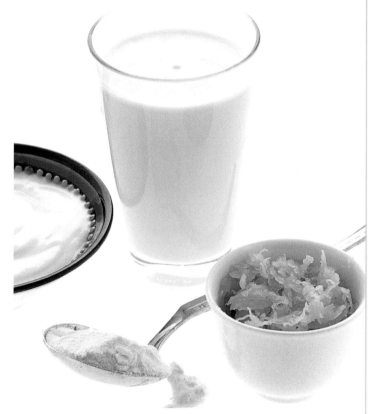

Above: Yoghurt, sauerkraut and whey are probiotics.
Below: Prebiotics include bananas and asparagus.

Are there tests for gut and liver function?
The normal liver function tests your doctor prescribes will pick up any raised liver enzymes, for example, in the case of alcohol excess. Specialized gut fermentation tests and liver toxicity tests are available at only a few laboratories.

People who have Gilbert's Syndrome will usually turn yellow if they fast for 24 to 36 hours. This is an inherited deficiency that is benign and does not require to be treated.

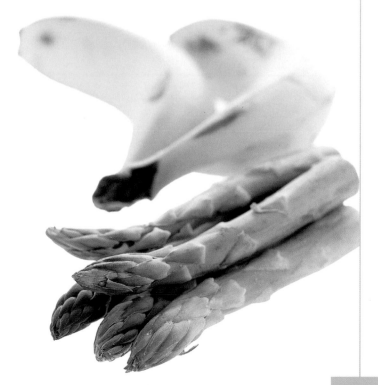

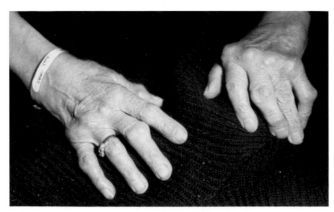

Osteoarthritis is a chronic degenerative disease in which free-radical attack and chronic inflammation both play a major role.

4 Chronic inflammation

Inflammation is part of the body's normal daily function. It is needed to repair damaged cells and fight foreign invading organisms. However, when the process goes out of control, it is not only damaged cells that are removed; healthy cells are also attacked and progressively destroyed. This leads to certain chronic diseases, including rheumatoid arthritis, multiple sclerosis, cancer, heart disease, inflammatory bowel disease and brain degeneration. Chronic inflammation accelerates ageing.

Soft, unstable material known as 'vulnerable plaque' is deposited inside blood vessels due to chronic inflammation and may break off, causing a heart attack.

What predisposes you to unbalanced inflammation?

(By 'unbalanced' we mean inflammation that is either excessive or insufficient.)

- A diet high in omega-6 essential fatty acids and low in omega-3 essential fatty acids. Fatty acids, derived from dietary fats, have many functions in the body. The two main groups, known as the omega-6 and omega-3 series, were well balanced in primitive man. However, with our increased intake of vegetable oils and margarine (which contains harmful transfatty acids), there is a predominance of omega-6 series, leading to chronic inflammation. On the other hand, the 'good' fatty acids such as the omega-3 flaxseed oil, linseed and fish oil, are beneficial, especially in the prevention of heart disease and stroke.
- Deficiencies of vitamins B6, B12 and folate may predispose you to high blood homocysteine levels, a risk factor for heart disease.
- A diet high in animal fats.
- Deficiencies of bioflavonoids and antioxidants found in fresh fruit and vegetables.
- Food additives, emulsifiers and flavouring agents. An example is tartrazine, which is a yellow colouring found in cheese, sweets and snacks.
- Benzoates, nitrates and sulphites, which are preservatives found in wine, beer, salads, cold meats, frozen chips, dried fruits and cold drinks.
- Monosodium glutamate (MSG), which is a popular flavour enhancer found in snack foods, peanuts, instant soups, soy sauce and Chinese food.
- Aspartame, an artificial sweetener found in soft drinks and diet foods. Aspartame and MSG are known as 'excitotoxins', which have an adverse effect on brain function.

It is therefore clear that unbalanced inflammation leads to premature ageing. The body's inflammatory processes need to be in balance for health and wellness. If they are underactive, you cannot fight infections or undertake tissue repair. If they are overactive, cells and tissues are damaged, resulting in auto-immune and degenerative diseases.

How can you keep inflammation balanced?

- Try to eat plenty of fish, especially sardines, herring, pilchards, anchovies, salmon trout and salmon.
- Add linseed to your morning cereal, or take flaxseed oil supplements.

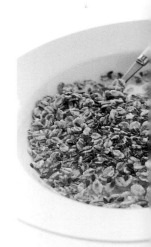

Right: Add linseed to your breakfast cereal to increase your omega-3 intake.

- Reduce animal fats and limit vegetable oils in your daily cooking. Avoid fried foods.
- Avoid processed or preserved foods, MSG and aspartame.
- Consume a variety of fruits and vegetables.

Are there tests for chronic inflammation?

Yes, there are specialized tests for estimating essential fatty acid profiles. CRP (cardio-reactive protein) is an essential test. Another test recommended as part of the cardiovascular profile is an estimation of homocysteine levels. A high homocysteine level is a risk factor for heart disease, and is associated with low levels of vitamins B6, B12 and folate. Supplementation with these vitamins will bring homocysteine levels back to normal and reduce your risk of heart disease.

5 A declining immune system

As you age, the immune systems normally begin to decline. Maintaining an efficient immune system is vital. A poorly functioning system not only accelerates ageing, it makes you vulnerable to carcinogens in the environment, bacteria and viruses, fungi and parasites, as well as a variety of diseases.

The immune system is your defence against foreign invaders. You have an army of specialized white blood cells, including so-called 'killer cells', that engulf and destroy bacteria, viruses and other unwanted foreign substances.

What are the signs when the immune system is not working?

- Frequent colds and flu
- Frequent chest infections and lingering sinusitis
- Candidiasis, or thrush
- Slow healing of wounds
- Recurring bacterial or viral infections

All these are signals indicating that you need to take action to improve your lifestyle and boost your immune system.

Right: Killer cells are specialized white blood cells that are part of your defence system to attack foreign invaders, such as bacteria, viruses and even cancer cells.

THE BODY'S LYMPHATIC SYSTEM

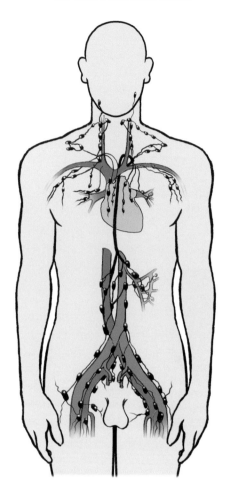

Hundreds of peripheral lymph nodes drain into larger lymph nodes situated along the major blood vessels.

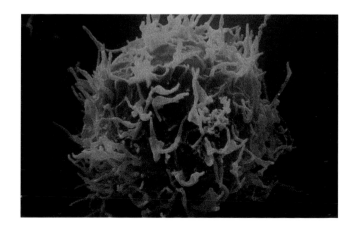

Can you boost immunity and maintain youthful levels?

- Correct nutrition is vital. Identify and replace allergenic foods.
- Limit intake of sugar in all its forms. Consuming 100g (3½ oz) of sugar (including fruit juice) will depress white cell and killer cell activity for one to five hours.
- Eat garlic and foods containing zinc or take zinc supplements.
- Supplement with antioxidants, vitamin C, vitamin E and co-enzyme Q10.
- Adaptogenic herbs are useful. Echinacea, astragalus, golden seal and shiitake mushrooms are well known. The Ayurvedic antioxidant, Amrit Kalash, and South African plant adaptogens, such as Sutherlandia and African potato (*Hypoxis rooperi*), are other supplements, now available internationally, that can be helpful. Sutherlandia has been used by indigenous people for centuries, and was dubbed the 'cancer bush' because of its use in aiding cancer patients. The African potato contains plant sterols and sterolins, which have been shown to help to boost immunity. It has also been used by traditional healers for centuries, but has only recently been researched at university level, and grown and produced with quality control.

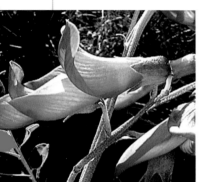

Sutherlandia

- Adopt stress-coping strategies and make sure you get adequate sleep and relaxation.
- Limit your use of antibiotics, steroids and anti-inflammatory drugs.
- Check your environment for air pollution, pesticides and heavy metals.

Is there a blood test for immune function?

The immune cell subset and tests for immunoglobulins are available, but a simple white cell count should be sufficient in most cases. This will be included in your basic blood profile.

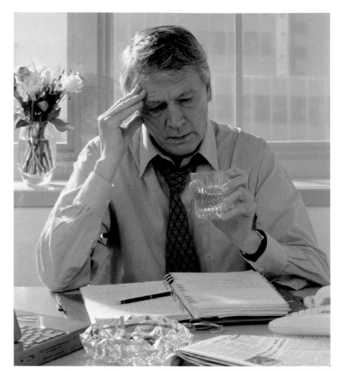

Chronic stress causes damage to the body's immune system, as well as to brain cells and hormones.

6 Prolonged stress

The hormone, cortisol, is produced by the adrenal glands in response to stress. Cortisol is necessary and in normal amounts is able to cope with everyday hassles as well as major life events that are stressful. If produced in excess over a period of time, however, it is extremely harmful and this can significantly accelerate ageing. To add to the problem, cortisol is the only steroid hormone that actually increases its levels as you age.

What are the harmful effects of excess cortisol?

- Most important is the fact that cortisol damages and actually kills brain cells. It is thus one of the factors increasing neurodegenerative conditions such as Alzheimer's disease and Parkinsonism.
- Cortisol depresses and damages your immune system, making you vulnerable to infections and even cancer.
- Excess cortisol also has an adverse effect on other hormones, such as insulin, thyroid and DHEA.

How can you lower stress hormones?

- Practise daily relaxation, meditation and mind-body therapies (*see* pages 100–101).
- Supplement your diet with 300mg magnesium daily, together with zinc, antioxidants and a cocktail of B vitamins.
- Supplement with herbal compounds known as adaptogens, which support the adrenal glands. These include Eleutherococcus (Siberian ginseng) and Sutherlandia. Eleutherococcus has been given to Russian athletes to improve stamina and endurance. Note that you should not take pure panax ginseng (also known as Chinese ginseng) as this can cause high blood pressure. Chinese doctors recommend its use only for patients who are debilitated. When panax ginseng is added to multiple formulas, it is only included in small amounts, and is thus not harmful.

- Consider taking DHEA (the adrenal prehormone, dehydroepiandrosterone) under medical supervision if your blood levels are below normal. Start with a small amount (5–25mg) and monitor your blood levels before and during supplementation. The action of DHEA includes its ability to balance cortisol and stress levels. DHEA also increases libido and generally improves your feeling of wellbeing.
- Pregnenalone is a precursor of DHEA, which is placed further up the hormone cascade. It is considered safer to use as an alternative to DHEA. Your doctor should supervise its use.

Are there tests to measure stress levels?

Yes, the adrenal stress index is a measurement of DHEA levels compared with cortisol levels. This blood test can be performed by your local laboratory.

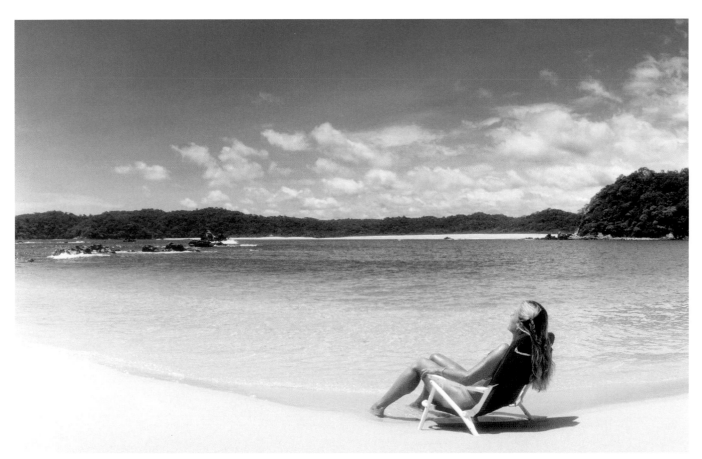

Go away now and again, and do nothing, for when you return your thoughts and perceptions will be clearer.

7 Waning hormones

The female menopause is associated with declining levels of DHEA, oestradiol, estrone, progesterone, melatonin and growth hormones. There is often a decrease in thyroid hormone as well. These changes begin during the perimenopause, which starts during a woman's late forties. Menopause starts at an average age of 50, with a dramatic drop in the female hormones oestradiol, estrone and progesterone.

The male menopause, known as the andropause, occurs gradually after the age of 50. Unlike the sudden drop of female hormones, the male hormone, testosterone, declines slowly. Symptoms of the andropause are often insidious and may be mistaken for depression and general fatigue.

Female hormones are responsible for urogenital health. Lack of these hormones after menopause may result in unpleasant symptoms, such as vaginal dryness and bladder discomfort with increased urination, which many women do not wish to discuss with their doctors. Oestrogen also benefits the skin, and helps preserve plumpness and integrity of the dermis.

Can you check for waning hormones?

Hormone profiles are easily obtained. Although most men do not consider having their hormones checked, it is advisable for men over 60, and those suffering from depression and fatigue, osteoporosis, or other symptoms of male menopause (*see* pages 56–57).

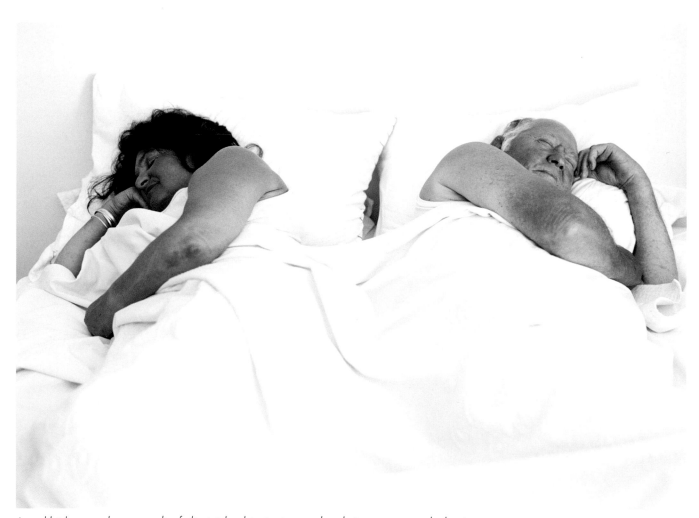

Low libido may be a result of diminished testosterone levels in men – and also in women.

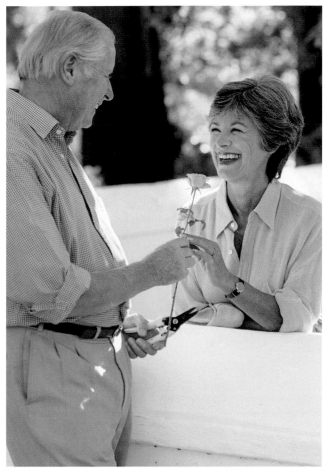

Multihormone replacement and herbal supplements can restore joie de vivre in both men and women.

How do you tackle declining hormones?

Multihormone replacement for both men and women has received much attention in recent years. Although it seems to be an attractive option, it is not without potentially dangerous side effects so it is essential that it should be monitored by your doctor. It is possible that in future each person could be prescribed an individualized transdermal skin patch containing a cocktail of hormones. With the current uncertainty regarding oestrogen and progesterone replacement therapy, many women prefer to go the 'natural' route. This involves the use of phyto- or plant oestrogens and herbs.

ACTION PLAN

➤ Implement baseline testing and laboratory tests after consulting your doctor. If you are unable to do comprehensive testing, do the basic essentials, including blood pressure, urine testing and blood sugar.

➤ Self-evaluation: look at your lifestyle, diet, habits and relationships, and how they affect your chronological age.

➤ Minimize the seven risk factors for premature ageing – starting today.

➤ Eat plenty of fresh fruit and vegetables containing antioxidants.

➤ Avoid refined carbohydrates such as white bread, cakes and sugar.

➤ Eat smaller, nutrient-dense meals.

➤ Do a modified fast one day a week.

➤ Supplement with omega-3 essential fatty acids and eat fish several times a week.

➤ Practise daily relaxation and meditation.

➤ Replace waning hormones with bio-identical hormones or use herbal supplements.

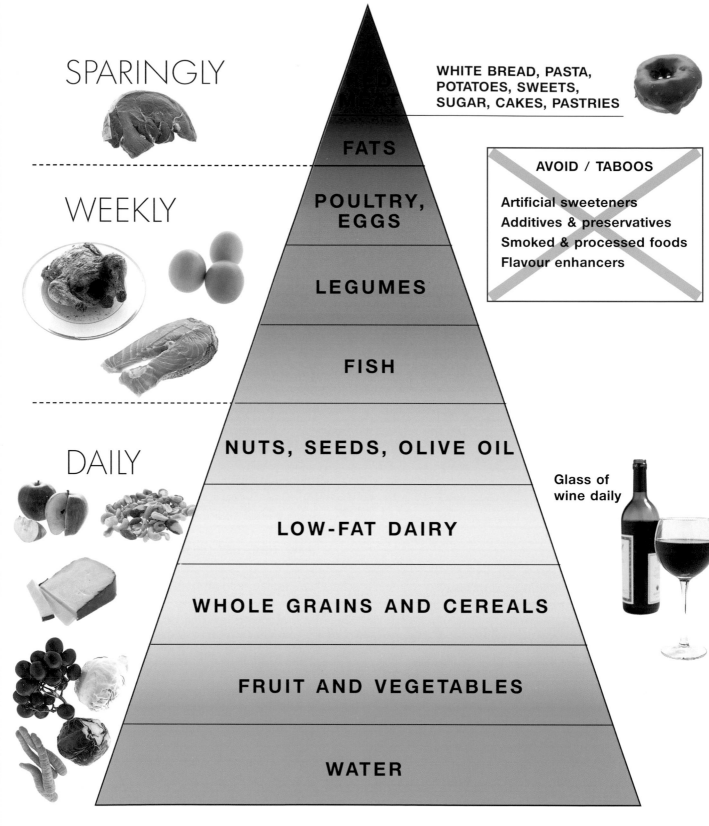

SPARINGLY

RED MEAT

WHITE BREAD, PASTA,
POTATOES, SWEETS,
SUGAR, CAKES, PASTRIES

FATS

WEEKLY

POULTRY, EGGS

AVOID / TABOOS

Artificial sweeteners
Additives & preservatives
Smoked & processed foods
Flavour enhancers

LEGUMES

FISH

DAILY

NUTS, SEEDS, OLIVE OIL

Glass of
wine daily

LOW-FAT DAIRY

WHOLE GRAINS AND CEREALS

FRUIT AND VEGETABLES

WATER

THE YOUTHFUL AGEING FOOD GUIDE PYRAMID

YOU ARE WHAT YOU EAT, ASSIMILATE AND ELIMINATE

Food can be either ageing or anti-ageing. It was Hippocrates who said, 'Let food be your medicine,' yet modern man seems to have forgotten the basic knowledge that, in fact, we are what we eat. The trillions of cells in our bodies depend on a daily meal of protein, fatty acids, carbohydrates and a cocktail of vitamins and minerals working together in synergy.

Yet each one of us is different. We are unique in terms of our individual rate of absorption, assimilation and dietary needs. The term used to describe this is 'biochemical individuality'.

Digestive problems are common in older people, and one of the most important contributing factors is dehydration. Although older people may feel less thirsty, dehydration is ageing. It shows up in the skin. Our bodies are composed of 70 per cent water, and many of our ailments are precipitated or aggravated by simple dehydration. Coffee, tea and alcohol are dehydrating, so they do not count in our daily fluid intake. We lose about two litres of fluid through respiration, and through our skin, kidneys and gut. This needs to be replaced daily.

Serial tea drinkers may develop zinc and iron deficiencies because absorption is blocked. A caffeine intake of more than 300mg daily – which is equivalent to two cups of strong coffee or three cups of tea – may cause headaches, indigestion and anxiety attacks, depending on the efficiency of an individual's liver's detoxification system.

What about alcohol? Is alcohol ageing? In fact, red wine in moderation is actually beneficial but remember that more than two drinks a day of any alcoholic beverage ages the skin, the arteries and just about every organ of the body.

We do not eat cigarettes, but it could be said that cigarettes eat us. Smoking is one of the worst culprits involved in skin ageing. Apart from being a serious risk factor for heart disease and cancer, smoking damages the collagen in our skin and causes premature wrinkles.

Foods that are anti-ageing are those that protect against cancer, heart disease and stroke, diabetes, high blood pressure, arthritis and most of the degenerative diseases. Ageing foods create free radicals and encourage rapid deterioration of body parts and functions.

An important research finding in recent years has been that calorie restriction prolongs life. In addition, we know that the metabolism slows down as we grow older, making it much easier to gain weight. The secret is to eat less, but choose nutrient-rich foods. If you think of the actual size of the stomach – which is about the size of a large grapefruit – it is easy to understand why it is advisable to limit the size of a meal to the amount that would fit into your outstretched palms.

The first thing you should do every morning is to look at your tongue, which is the gateway to and monitor of your digestive system. It should be smooth and glossy rather than furry and a greenish-grey colour.

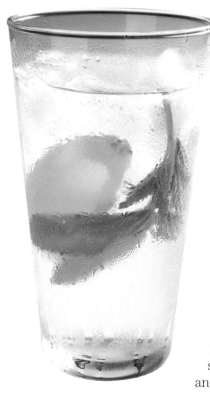

Drink six to eight glasses of water daily.

FOODS THAT AGE	FOODS THAT PROTECT AND REVITALIZE
Animal fats, saturated fats	Freshly squeezed vegetable juice
Trans-fatty acids, e.g. margarine	Sprouts and seeds (e.g. pumpkin, linseed)
Fried foods, roasts and barbecues	Red grapes
Rancid nuts and oils	Yoghurt, fermented foods
Smoked and salted products	Tomatoes, cruciferous vegetables
Processed meats, salami, sausage	Garlic, turmeric and ginger
White bread, cakes and biscuits	Sardines, salmon and fatty fish
Sugar, sweets	Soy products, tofu
Additives and preservatives	Sea vegetables
Excitotoxins, e.g. aspartame	Wheat grass, barley grass, spirulina
Monosodium glutamate	Olive oil
Excessive alcohol	Beetroot
Overeating	Blueberries, cherries

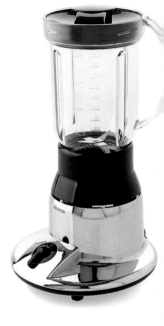

JUICING AND SHAKING

Everyone should have a juice extractor machine and/or blender in the kitchen. Making freshly processed vegetable and fruit juices will provide you with living plant enzymes, phytonutrients and easily absorbed vitamins and minerals.

There are many different combinations, and you can experiment with a variety of fruit and vegetables for a great way to start the day.

ANTI-AGEING REVITAJUICE

Combine in a juice extractor:

4–6 carrots

2 sticks of celery

half a beetroot

0.5cm fresh ginger root

a sprinkling of wheat grass

and/or alfalfa sprouts

125ml (4 fl oz) water

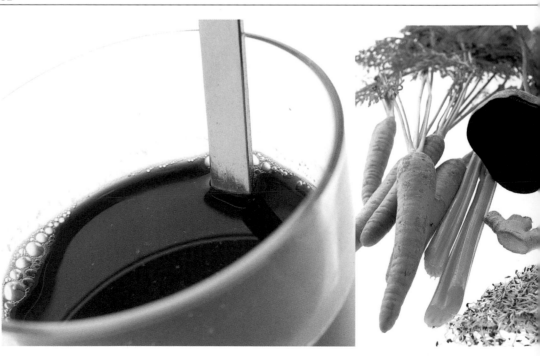

Use a blender to make the Supershake below for breakfast or for a snack later in the day. Soya milk is readily available either dried in powder form or as a liquid in cartons. It is an excellent source of isoflavones for women, with the added benefit of improving bone density.

SUPERSHAKE

Blend together:

250ml (½ pt) soya milk

1 banana or some strawberries

1 Tbsp honey

1 Tbsp wheatgerm

1 tsp sesame seeds

1 tsp sunflower seeds

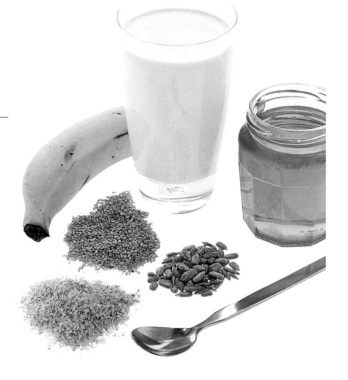

Do you chew food 30 times before swallowing? Food needs to be mixed thoroughly with alkaline salivary juices in the mouth before reaching the stomach, where acid gastric juices begin their work. The food-combining theory of separating starches and proteins has not been proved scientifically, but it is a fact that older people especially benefit from this practice. Raw fruit should be eaten separately because it will ferment and cause bloating if eaten with cooked food. The best time to eat fruit is mid-morning, mid-afternoon and as a snack.

LOW STOMACH ACID

Once food has left the stomach, it enters the duodenum and small intestine, where it is tackled by the digestive enzymes lipase protease and amylase. Older people are often deficient in these enzymes, as well in gastric juices. More than 50 per cent of

people over 60 have low stomach acidity, resulting in bloating, indigestion and chronic gut problems.

A simple way to determine whether you have low stomach acid is to take a teaspoonful of apple cider vinegar in some water. If this makes your heartburn go away, then you need more gastric acid, so you may then take a little apple cider vinegar in water before meals. If it makes your symptoms worse, however, then you have too much acidity and you should not take digestive enzymes that contain hydrochloric acid (HCl). Betaine HCl, for example, is included in many digestive aids.

With ageing, digestive problems may result in excessive gas, bloating, constipation or diarrhoea. In addition, nutritional deficiencies may develop due to inadequate absorption of nutrients, especially vitamin B12, calcium, iron, zinc and protein. Some 20 to 30 per cent of older people develop atrophy of the stomach lining, leading to inadequate amounts of gastric juices. Combined with diminished production of digestive enzymes, plus damage to the gut lining, this is bad news for nutrient absorption.

Taking antacids for indigestion will neutralize stomach acids and interfere with digestion. Many antacids also contain aluminium, which is toxic in large amounts and is also thought to be a factor in Alzheimer's disease.

What are the symptoms of low stomach acid?
- Dilated veins on cheeks and nose
- Bloating and belching immediately after eating
- Feeling excessively full after meals
- Indigestion
- Weak, peeling or cracked fingernails
- Rectal itching
- Chronic gut problems, e.g. Candida

LEAKY GUT
With assimilation and absorption taking place in the small and large intestines, it is essential to keep these organs healthy. Apart from factors that can damage the gut, such as toxins in foods, ageing in itself is associated with altered intestinal permeability and the possibility of developing what is commonly known as 'the leaky gut syndrome'. When this happens, abnormal proteins and molecules of food are leaked through the cell junctions into the bloodstream, causing a heavy load on the liver.

What causes a leaky gut?
- Incorrect diet, food allergies, poor digestion
- Alcohol in excess
- Stress
- Antibiotics, anti-inflammatory drugs, hormones
- Ageing
- Decreased immunity
- The 'Hoover syndrome' or overeating

What symptoms are associated with a leaky gut?
- Feeling generally unwell, 'vertically ill', fatigue, headaches
- Joint and muscle pains
- Skin rashes, allergies
- Chemical sensitivities
- Fatigue when exercising
- Brain fogging, inability to concentrate

IMPROVE DIGESTION AND NUTRIENT ABSORPTION
1. Eat mindfully, consider the nutrients that you are consuming, chew food thoroughly, and preferably choose unprocessed, organically grown foods. Colour-code your plate with a combination of orange, yellow, green and red vegetables.
2. Start each day with a glass of hot water and lemon. Do not drink with meals as this dilutes the alkaline salivary juices.
3. Herbal bitters – for example, Schweden bitters – stimulate the stomach to produce gastric juices. Half to one teaspoonful in a little water can be taken with meals.
4. Eat less at mealtimes but have a mid-morning and mid-afternoon snack.
5. Daily exercise will help to improve both your metabolism and digestion.
6. Zinc deficiency is often related to inadequate digestion in older people, especially those who drink tea. You can supplement with 15–20mg zinc piccolinate daily, taken at night.
7. Have a modified fast (*see* page 36) once a week.
8. Detoxify your system for one week every three to four months (*see* page 37).

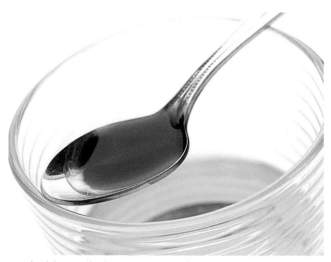

Herbal bitters help to improve digestion.

DETOXIFICATION

In order to run smoothly, your car needs regular servicing and maintenance, including a radiator flush and change of spark plugs. Although our bodies are generally self-servicing, small, degenerative changes occur as we grow older. Moreover, ageing is associated with impaired detoxification processes. It is not normal to have indigestion, constipation, aches and pains, headaches or fatigue. When your liver is not functioning properly you will feel sluggish and possibly nauseous. Your eyes can be affected by the liver in many ways: for instance, bloodshot eyes may mirror the condition of an overloaded liver.

Many diseases – including cancer, auto-immune disorders such as rheumatoid arthritis, and brain degenerative disorders – are associated with poor liver function.

What causes poor liver function?
- Accumulated toxins such as alcohol and caffeine
- Incorrect diet, additives and preservatives, colouring agents, excessive animal fats, trans-fatty acids
- Overeating: the liver absorbs food like a sponge
- Medications such as analgesics and anti-inflammatory drugs

The role of the liver in detoxification
Every substance that is absorbed by the intestines must first pass through the liver before going on to the general circulation. The liver is the major organ of detoxification and your health and energy are largely dependent on its efficiency. It disposes of a daily dose of toxins produced internally from bowel contents, food, water and medications, and externally from the air you breathe.

Right: The tongue is the gateway to the digestive system.

THE DIGESTIVE SYSTEM

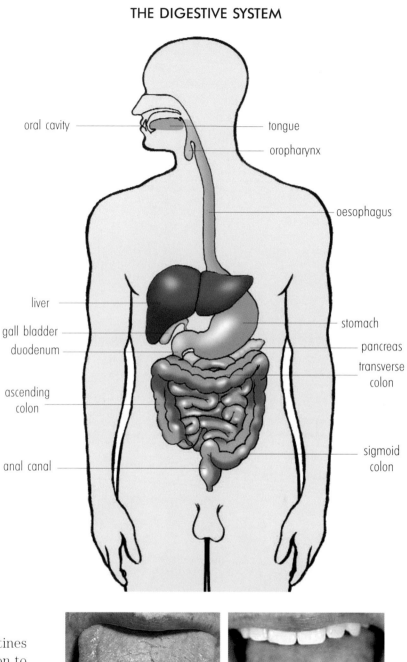

oral cavity
tongue
oropharynx
oesophagus
liver
gall bladder
duodenum
stomach
pancreas
transverse colon
ascending colon
sigmoid colon
anal canal

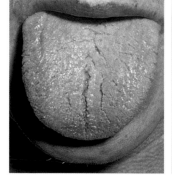

TOXIC TONGUE

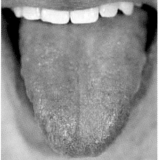

HEALTHY TONGUE

One-day modified fast

Implementing a modified fast one day a week will help to lessen the load on the liver and gut, and is a painless procedure.

During the day drink only filtered water and herb tea, and eat fresh fruit such as papaya, but exclude bananas, grapefruit and melon. For supper make a vegetable soup or consommé.

POTATO PEELING BROTH

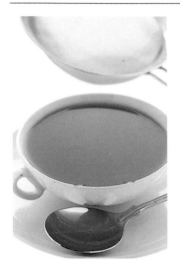

3 potatoes, cut in half
1 carrot, sliced
1 celery stalk
½ onion
750ml (1½ pt) water

Cut the peel from the potatoes, keeping 1cm of potato with the peel. Discard potato centre. Add peel to vegetables and water. Cook for 30 minutes. Strain and drink the broth.

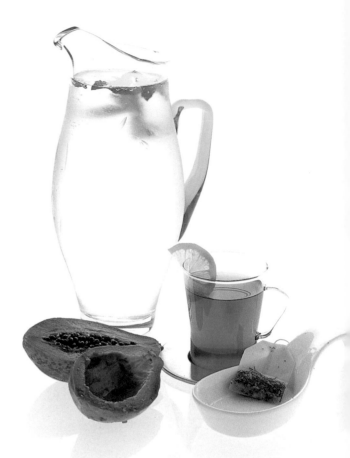

During a one-day modified fast, enjoy herbal tea and drink plenty of water. Eat fruit such as papaya during the day, and make a vegetable soup for supper.

A longer detox programme can be undertaken every three to four months, resulting in a tremendous feeling of wellbeing and vitality. It will improve digestion, revitalize the liver, and slow down degenerative changes throughout your body. Overeating is the most common cause of liver malfunction.

Remember the concept of biochemical individuality and the fact that we are all different, and have different needs. You should not fast or detoxify if you are suffering from a debilitating illness or from kidney disease.

Prolonged fasting as a means of weight reduction is not recommended because you will lose lean body mass and thus slow down your metabolic rate, making it more difficult to lose weight.

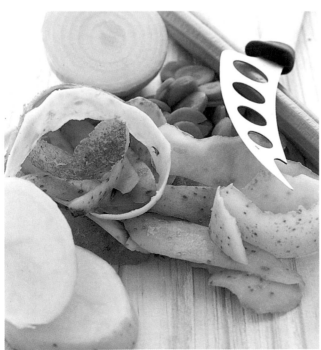

Left: Potatoes, carrots, celery and onion are boiled up together to make a detoxifying broth.

Seven-day detox programme

1. For the week before your detox, gradually reduce your caffeine intake. If you stop it suddenly, you may experience withdrawal symptoms, such as nausea, headache and muscular pain.

2. The evening before you start, take a laxative such as cascara or a small amount of Epsom salts. Obviously, omit this if you have colitis or any inflammatory bowel problems. For supper, have a light meal of vegetable soup.

3. For the duration of your detox programme, start the day with a glass of hot water and lemon, and drink at least six glasses of water during the day. Adding herbs such as mint and fennel creates interest. If you prefer hot drinks, rooibos/redbush tea with a slice of lemon is a relaxing antioxidant.

4. **Days 1 and 2.** Choose either fruit only (excluding grapefruit and bananas) or vegetable juices and strained vegetable broth. Note that grapefruit and grapefruit juice contain the compound naringenin, which inhibits liver detoxification. Bananas should be excluded because they have a high concentration of carbohydrates and are not a juicy fruit, which is preferable.

5. **Days 3 to 5. Breakfast:** choose two or three fruits (excluding grapefruit and banana).
   Lunch and supper: choose either a mixed raw salad, or stir-fried or steamed vegetables. At one of these meals, include a baked potato. At the other, choose from either 125g (4½ oz) of low-fat cottage cheese or one hardboiled or poached egg.
   Snacks: 125ml (4½ oz) plain, low-fat yoghurt or an apple or pear mid-morning and mid-afternoon.

6. **Days 6 and 7. Breakfast:** Soak muesli in a bowl of water overnight. Add grated, peeled apple, together with 125g low-fat, plain yoghurt.
   Mid-morning: fruit.
   Lunch and supper: at one meal choose a mixed salad with baked potato, cottage cheese, and one or two slices of wholewheat or rye bread. For the other meal choose either fish or chicken or tofu, together with mixed vegetables.

7. Daily skin brushing with a soft, dry brush before bathing, as well as massage and hydrotherapy, help to aid lymphatic drainage during detoxification. Sauna helps to remove toxins from the fatty tissue. The lymphatic system consists of a comprehensive network of lymph vessels throughout the body, with a chain of superficial lymph glands draining into deep lymph nodes following major blood vessels. Lymphatics form a major pathway for the elimination of toxins and waste products draining into the blood circulation.

8. Liver function may be supported by including beetroot – raw, cooked or juiced – in your diet. A really good vegetable juice combination would include beetroot, carrots and celery. Herbal supplements such as milk thistle, dandelion and artichoke will be discussed later (*see* page 51).

9. Alpha lipoic acid is an especially good antioxidant, which has a beneficial effect in helping to remove toxins from the liver.

At the end of your detoxification programme you should both look and feel years younger.

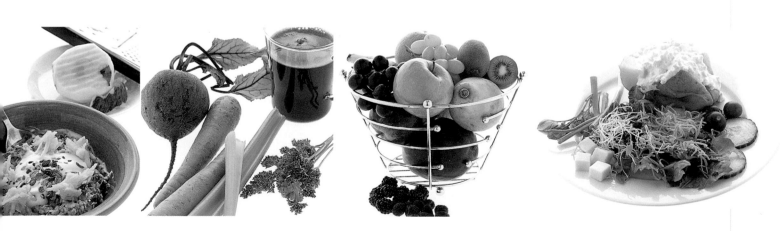

FIGHT CANCER WITH KNIFE AND FORK

We have come a long way in our understanding of cancer, but still a final solution eludes us. Cancer is one of the top three causes of death in older people, and as we are living longer, we should do all we can to prevent this most sinister of diseases. It is encouraging to know that we have the ability to do something to help prevent it. At least 35 per cent of all cancers are associated with incorrect diet and, in the case of colon cancer, diet may account for 80 per cent of cases. The most common cancer in women is breast cancer. In men, prostate cancer incidence equals that of breast cancer in women.

How does cancer develop?

We know that three stages result in an explosion of uncontrolled cell growth and tumour formation. The first stage involves a reaction between the cancer-producing substance (carcinogen) and the DNA of cells in a particular organ. There may be a genetic susceptibility. This stage may remain dormant, and the individual may only be at risk for developing cancer at a later stage.

The second stage of cancer growth occurs very slowly over a period that can range from several months to as much as 20 or 30 years. During this stage, a change in diet and lifestyle can have such a beneficial effect that the person may not develop cancer during his or her lifetime.

The third and final stage involves progression and spread of the cancer, at which point changes in diet may have less of an impact. Carcinogens in the diet that trigger off the DNA cell changes include moulds and aflatoxins (for example, in peanuts and maize), nitrosamines (in smoked meats and other cured products), rancid fats and cooking oils, alcohol, additives and preservatives. The weekend barbecue is not so healthy either. Compounds known as heterocyclic amines form on the surface of the meat while it is grilling, and these are known to be carcinogenic. A combination of foods may have a cumulative effect, and when incorrect diet is added to other risk factors such as a polluted environment, smoking, ultraviolet radiation, free radicals, lack of exercise, and stress, the stage is set for DNA damage and cancer progression.

CANCER TRIGGERS

- Moulds and aflatoxins in foods
- Nitrosamines in smoked meats, salamis, preserved and cured products
- Barbecued meats
- Rancid fats and cooking oils
- Additives and preservatives
- Excessive amounts of animal fats
- Environmental pollution and ultraviolet radiation
- Incorrect diet, with smoking or lack of exercise
- Stress

The role of diet in preventing cancer

There is a great deal of scientific research that emphasizes the role of diet in both the causation and prevention of cancer. Professor Walter Willet from the Harvard School of Public Health states, 'Ongoing research continues to support the view that diet significantly influences the incidence of many human cancers.' He goes on to recommend that in addition to correct diet, a daily multivitamin supplement containing folic acid should be taken.

What foods protect against cancer?

1. Vegetables, especially cruciferous vegetables – broccoli, cabbage, brussel sprouts and cauliflower – reduce the risk of prostate cancer. A US study was conducted on newly diagnosed prostate cancer patients who were then placed on a trial of fruit and vegetables for five years. It was found that while fruit was not protective, cruciferous vegetables did reduce the risk of cancer progression. Other foods with a beneficial effect on prostate health include: tomatoes, which contain lycopene, and plant sterols found in pumpkin seeds, the African potato and some vegetables.
2. A study involving 35,000 non-smoking, mainly vegetarian, Seventh Day Adventists found a reduced risk of lung, prostate, pancreatic and colon cancers. They also had a 25 per cent lower incidence

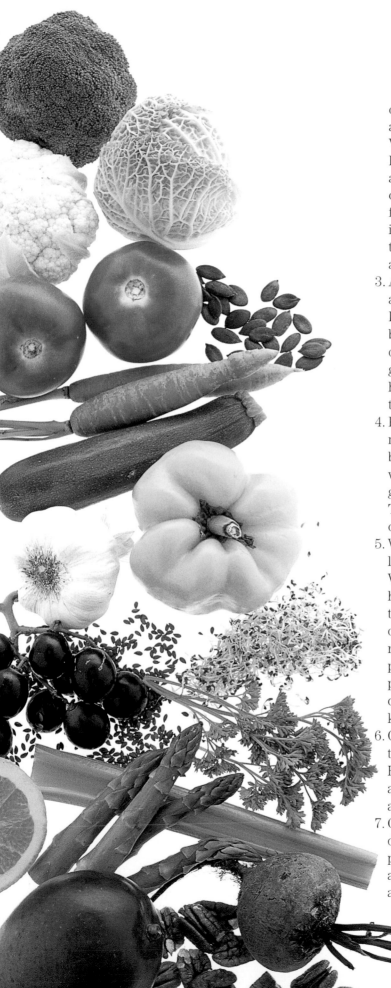

of diabetes, high blood pressure and arthritis, and a 30 per cent reduced risk of heart disease. Vegetarians have a reduced risk of most cancers. Fruit and vegetables contain the antioxidant vitamins A, C and E, as well as many other anti-cancer ingredients such as selenium, fibre, flavonoids, indoles, phenols, carotenoids, sterols, isoflavones, anthocyanidins and resveratrol. From this list it would seem to be reasonable to include a wide variety of vegetables in the diet.

3. Antioxidants found in fruit and vegetables protect against both stomach and large bowel cancer. In India, the low incidence of large bowel cancer can be attributed to a diet that is high in carbohydrates and natural antioxidants, such as turmeric, garlic and ginger. Garlic, in particular, is known to have antibacterial and antifungal properties, and to promote a healthy gastrointestinal tract.

4. Probiotics, including yoghurt, whey and fermented foods such as sauerkraut, contain lactobacilli, bifidobacteria and acidophilus bacteria, which help to counteract overgrowth of harmful gut bacteria and provide a healthy gut milieu. This, in turn, helps to prevent the start of colon cancer and other bowel cancers.

5. Women in Japan and the Far East have a much lower incidence of breast cancer than those in the West. In addition to a high vegetable intake they have a high consumption of soy products containing isoflavones, which are plant or phyto-oestrogens. Phyto-oestrogens bind the oestrogen receptors in the body and block the cancer-promoting effects of oestrogen. In addition to soy, plant oestrogens are found in red clover, black cohosh, rhubarb, alfalfa and linseed (which is also known as flaxseed).

6. Grapes have strong antioxidant properties in the seeds and pith, which contain quercitin. Resveratrol, which is found in red grape skins, also has anticancer properties and helps to protect against heart disease.

7. Cancer is linked to a poorly functioning liver detoxification system. Healthy liver function is promoted by the herbs dandelion, milk thistle and artichoke. Beetroot is particularly beneficial and may be eaten raw, cooked or juiced. Raw

vegetable juices, including carrots, celery and parsley, together with beetroot, are an excellent way of providing concentrated antioxidants and plant enzymes. Wheat grass is easily grown at home and may be included in juices or perhaps sprinkled on salads. To promote liver detoxification you should eat plenty of cruciferous vegetables and foods rich in vitamin B (e.g. whole grains and cereals), and vitamin C (e.g. cabbage, broccoli and brussel sprouts, sweet peppers, oranges and tangerines). Citrus is beneficial but avoid grapefruit, as it contains naringenin, which may inhibit detoxification of the liver by up to 30 per cent. Glutathione-rich foods, such as avocado, asparagus and walnuts, are also good for detoxifying the liver.

Liver protectors include:
- Dandelion (*Taraxacum*)
- Milk thistle (*Silybum*)
- Artichoke (*Cynara*)
- Beetroot – raw, juiced or cooked
- Wheat grass
  - Cruciferous vegetables
    - Avocado
    - Asparagus
    - Walnuts

8. Together with a healthy liver, a healthy intestine is critical for cancer prevention. Improving your digestion, avoiding constipation, and consuming probiotics, plenty of fibre, as well as antioxidants, are all part of the overall plan. To reach the recommended 30g (1oz) of fibre per day, you need to eat the equivalent of four slices of bread, a bowl of breakfast oats, as well as five fruits and vegetables.

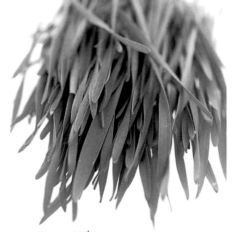
Wheat grass

9. Squalene found in olive oil has been shown in animal studies to inhibit colon, lung and skin cancers.
10. A new anticancer compound, as yet unnamed, has recently been found in mangoes. Mangoes, as with all yellow fruits and vegetables, also contain cancer-preventing carotenoids.

To summarize:
1. Eat at least five portions of fruit and vegetables daily, ensuring that you choose a wide variety. Try to include some cruciferous vegetables (examples include brussel sprouts, cabbage, cauliflower and broccoli), a leafy green vegetable, a red fruit or vegetable, as well as either yellow or orange vegetables or fruit.
2. Eat more fibre in wholegrain cereals, fruit and vegetables to improve bowel transit time and promote a healthy gut environment.
3. Avoid processed meat, and smoked and salted products. Cut down on roasts and barbecues.

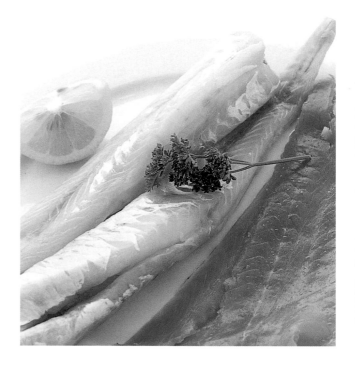

Left: Olive oil, a monounsaturated fat, may inhibit colon, lung and skin cancers.
Right: Include plenty of fish in your diet.

4. Avoid rancid fats in cooking oils, and transfatty acids in margarine.
5. Eat more omega-3 rich fish, especially fatty fish.
6. Avoid additives and preservatives by reading all food labels carefully.
7. Avoid plastic wrapping (which contains oestrogen-like compounds), and do not use aluminium cooking utensils.
8. Food should be fresh in order to avoid ingesting moulds and aflatoxins.
9. The cumulative effect of inappropriate foods, together with smoking, excess alcohol, obesity and lack of exercise, can trigger cancer.
10. Stress depletes the immune system and decreases the activity of natural killer cells. During times of stress it is vital that you should concentrate on an optimum cancer-protecting diet, and on taking additional antioxidant and multi-vitamin supplements.
11. In addition to diet, follow the general rules of a healthy lifestyle, especially exercise. The incidence of colon cancer has been shown to be inversely related to exercise.

ACTION PLAN

➤ Revise your diet. Choose foods that increase vitality and prevent cancer, heart disease and degenerative disorders. Try to arrange a rainbow of five different colours on your plate.

➤ Eat less, but drink more water. Eat mindfully and chew thoroughly.

➤ Improve your digestion, gut and liver function. Take supplements, if appropriate.

➤ Detox regularly. Eliminate toxins from your diet, your environment and your emotions.

➤ Take care of your skin. Nourish from within, hydrate and protect.

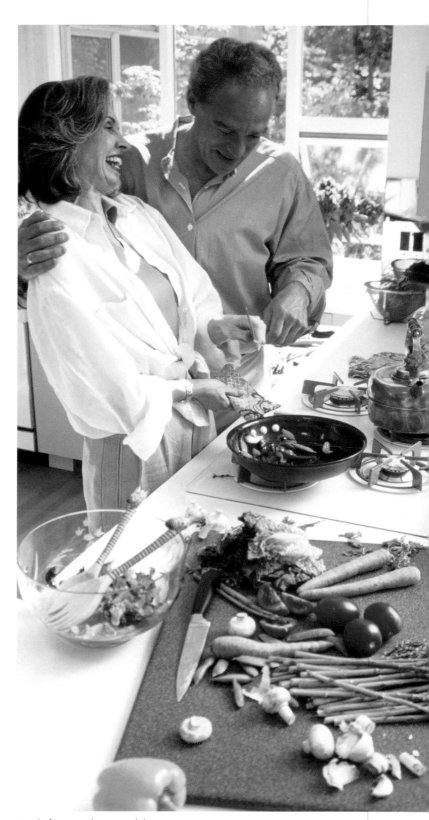

Fresh fruit and vegetables are easy to prepare.

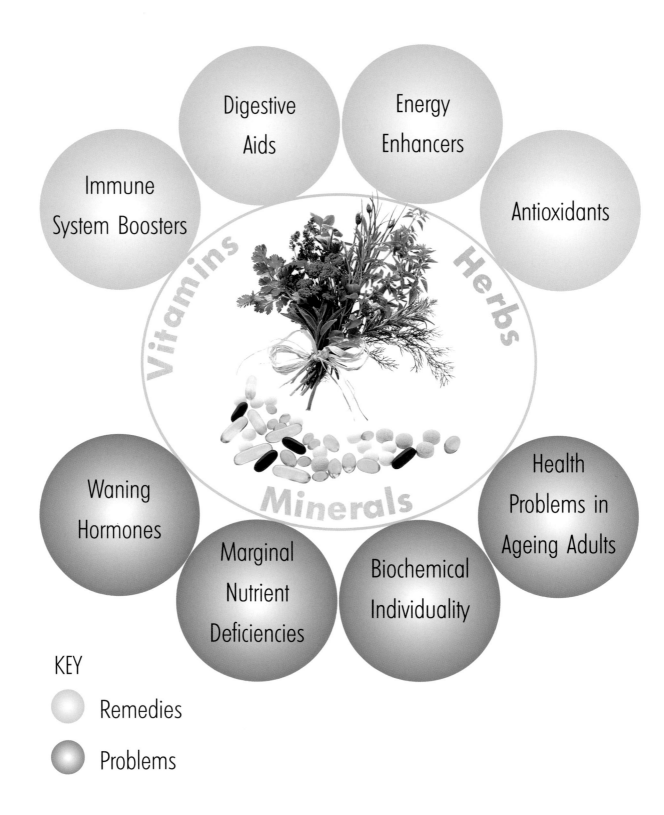

Digestive Aids

Energy Enhancers

Immune System Boosters

Antioxidants

Vitamins

Herbs

Minerals

Waning Hormones

Health Problems in Ageing Adults

Marginal Nutrient Deficiencies

Biochemical Individuality

KEY

Remedies

Problems

VITAMINS, MINERALS AND HERBAL SUPPLEMENTS

Why do older people need nutritional supplements? We often hear the comments, 'If I eat a balanced diet surely I will get all the vitamins and minerals I need?' or 'Taking extra vitamins will give you expensive urine.' The fact is that very few of us eat a truly balanced diet.

Do you eat at least five fruits and vegetables every day? Food preparation has changed dramatically since the days of our ancestors. We are now eating more convenience foods, which contain additives and preservatives, colouring agents and flavour enhancers. Hopefully, after you read this book you will take care with your food choices and look for organic fruit and vegetables grown without herbicides and pesticides. You will also eat unprocessed and unrefined food.

There is another problem. After many years of cultivation our soil has become depleted of nutrients. A carrot that contained 12 per cent magnesium 20 years ago now contains only 3 per cent when it is grown in the same patch of soil.

With ageing comes impaired absorption of nutrients for a variety of reasons – inadequate digestion due to the inability to chew properly (dental problems), low stomach acid, low digestive enzymes, a leaky gut due to medications, excessive tea drinking, as well as the inherent problem of an ageing gut.

In today's environment we are bombarded with free radicals, which cause premature ageing. This makes it important for us to defend ourselves with an adequate intake of antioxidants.

We are all familiar with the antioxidants vitamin A, betacarotene, vitamins C and E. However, there are many other antioxidants in fruit and vegetables, and they all combat free radical attack. Some of the most useful are the flavonoids (found in citrus, sweet peppers and other vegetables), pycnogenol (from pine bark and grape seeds) and lycopene (in tomatoes). Recent research has also succeeded in identifying several other age-defying antioxidants.

ANTIOXIDANTS FOR THE 21ST CENTURY
Resveratrol
The grape diet is used as a cleansing and elimination diet, and as a means of providing a hefty dose of antioxidants. The 'French paradox' refers to the fact that the average French person consumes above-average quantities of red wine and plenty of fatty cheese, yet has a low incidence of heart disease. The secret appears to be the grapes from which wine is made. The grape seed contains pycnogenol, the flesh of the grape contains vitamin C, and the skin of red grapes contains resveratrol. Resveratrol has anticancer, anti-inflammatory and strong antioxidant properties. It has been shown to be effective in the prevention of atherosclerosis (hardening of the arteries) and heart disease. You may take resveratrol in supplement form, or you may enjoy eating red grapes and drinking red wine (in moderation, of course). Long-distance travellers may take resveratrol one hour before and every four hours during a flight or car journey to reduce the risk of deep-vein thrombosis.

Alpha lipoic acid (ALA)
This is a naturally occurring co-enzyme in our bodies, which is involved in all the energy processes. It is a potent antioxidant and unique in that it is both fat and water soluble.

Red grapes contain antioxidants.

ALA acts synergistically with vitamins C and E, enhancing their actions. ALA thus guards against numerous degenerative diseases and slows down the ageing process. It protects the brain cells and the liver, and protects against 'AGEs' or protein glycosylation (*see* page 21). It is useful for diabetics in helping to control unstable blood sugar levels. It is also available in some of the latest cosmetics and is used in the treatment of skin photo-ageing. Can we find ALA in our food? Yes, but only in small amounts in foods such as kidneys, red meat, spinach and broccoli. To be effective, it should be taken as a supplement in amounts of 50–100mg per day.

Melatonin

This remarkable hormone, produced by the pineal gland, not only works as a sleeping aid, but is a potent antioxidant, immune booster and guardian of our ageing clock. It is produced in the dark while

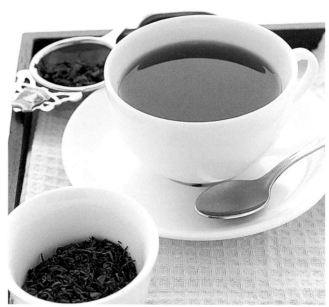

Green tea is a healthy beverage with strong antioxidant properties. It helps to prevent cancer, protects the heart and can lower blood sugar levels.

you sleep. If you get up during the night and put on a bright light, melatonin production stops immediately. Low melatonin levels are associated with premature ageing. We know that seven hours' sleep a night in a darkened room is anti-ageing, whereas insomnia or lack of sleep is ageing. Leading Swiss researcher Professor Walter Pierpoli was able to extend the lifespan of mice by 20 per cent using melatonin. Supplementation with melatonin is still controversial, but if you decide to take it, start with the lowest possible dose (1–3mg) taken half an hour before bedtime on alternate days. Melatonin production declines with age, so supplementation may be beneficial after the age of 50.

Green tea extract

Green tea is made from the plant *Camellia sinensis*. It contains polyphenols and bioflavonoids that have anticancer properties and protect the heart and blood vessels against free radical attack. Green tea is an antioxidant that also helps to lower blood sugar levels, so it is useful for diabetics and in weight loss programmes.

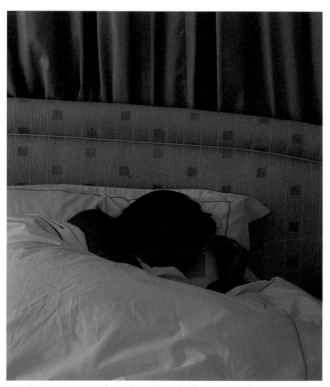

Melatonin is produced in the dark as you sleep.

Proanthocyanidins

Also known by the name pycnogenol, proanthocyanidins are antioxidants that are extracted from pine bark and grape seed. They can be useful in helping to treat arthritis and other degenerative disorders, including vascular problems such as varicose veins, spider veins and poor circulation.

Co-enzyme Q10

Co-enzyme Q10 is found in small quantities in most foods, but can also be taken as a supplement. Research has found it to be useful when combined with other supplements in the treatment of angina and heart disease, as well as other degenerative disorders, including periodontal (gum) disease. In older persons it helps to increase energy levels and stimulate the immune system.

Carnosine

Carnosine is an amino acid with strong antioxidant properties. This supplement is helpful in the prevention of cataracts and degenerative diseases, such as Alzheimer's disease and Parkinsonism. Russian researchers have developed carnosine eyedrops, which are being used for age-related eye disorders. Carnosine should not be confused with either carnitine or acetyl-l carnitine, which are also amino acids.

GETTING ENOUGH NUTRIENTS

How do you know if nutrients are not at optimal levels in your diet? You can have a blood test done by a specialized laboratory, or you can also check symptoms of deficiency that may apply to you. Described below are three nutrients that are often suboptimal, and therefore contribute to premature ageing.

Do you need magnesium?

Signs include:
* Muscle cramps in legs or feet
* Muscle twitches
* Aching muscles
* Migraine headaches
* Dental pain
* Brain 'fogging'
* Anxiety or irritability
* Restless legs

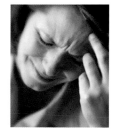

Migraine

Do you need essential fatty acids?

Signs include:
* 'Chicken skin' or goose bumps on the back of the arms
* Unusual thirst
* Joint stiffness or pain
* Dry eyes
* Soft, flaking or brittle nails
* Frequent urination
* Premenstrual breast pain
* Dry, cracked skin on heels

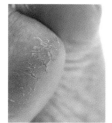

Cracked heels

Do you need zinc?

Signs include:
* White spots on fingernails
* Poor smell or taste
* Slow wound healing
* Frequent infections
* Sugar craving
* Stretch marks

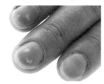

Spots on fingernails

SUPPLEMENTATION POINTERS

Before you start taking supplements, you need to remember the following points.
* Extra vitamins and minerals are only as good as the diet accompanying them.
* To ensure that supplements are absorbed, your digestive tract and liver need to be healthy.
* Supplementation with nutrients will not give you a 'quick fix'. Take them regularly for at least three months in order to see benefits, which may be subtle.
* When taking vitamins and minerals you should have a 'wash out' period every three or four months. Stop taking them while you practise your seven-day detoxifying programme to give the bowel a rest and clean out any debris.
* Remember the concept of biochemical individuality: each of us is different, we have different requirements, and we absorb and utilize nutrients differently.
* Vitamin E has several

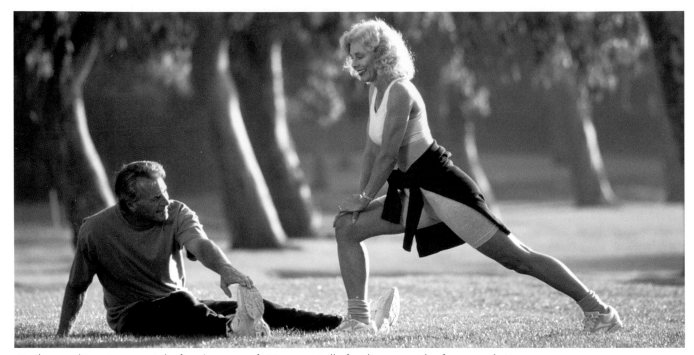

Daily stretching is essential after the age of 40, especially for those at risk of osteoarthritis.

forms, with the most common one being alpha-tocopherol. The most potent form is tocotrienol, so look for this in your vitamin E supplement.

• Water-soluble vitamins such as vitamin C and the B group are best taken in a slow-release form. The body has limited storage capacity and excess will be eliminated in the urine if they are taken in bulk.

There is a vast amount of information on the topic of supplementation. This book focuses on the most common health problems associated with ageing, and suggests herbs, vitamins and minerals, as well as natural therapies, to protect against, alleviate and reduce underlying pathology. Some of the supplements will have recommended amounts, but others depend on the actual product, which has varying amounts according to the manufacturer's formula.

ARTHRITIS
Osteoarthritis
This is a degenerative disorder that is put down to wear and tear of joints, but there is a great deal that you can do to prevent or reduce this most common problem of ageing.

Diet, as in everything else, is vital. Avoid acid-forming foods, especially wheat, animal products and sugar. Drink more water and detox regularly. The cartilage surfaces of bones in each joint contain water that acts as lubrication when two opposing surfaces glide over each other during movement. When you are dehydrated, lubrication is impaired. This results in pain signals and swelling of the joint, with ultimate breakdown or erosion of cartilage.

Daily stretching and back exercises should be part of everyone's regime, and is essential after the age of 40. Hydrotherapy (*see* pages 65–68) and gentle exercise in a heated pool (*see* page 91) are excellent for anyone with joint pains or stiffness.

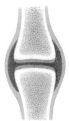 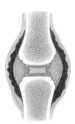 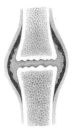

healthy knee joint   *rheumatoid arthritis*   *osteoarthritis*

Supplements:
1. Pycnogenol pine bark extract, 30–100mg daily
2. Vitamin E, 400 units daily
3. Essential fatty acids, especially salmon oil
4. Glucosamine, chondroitin and MSM (methyl-sulfonyl-methane), which is a nonmetallic sulphur compound, in combination
5. Calcium, magnesium and boron combination

Other supplements that may be useful (bearing biochemical individuality in mind) are New Zealand green-lipped mussel, sea cucumber and cetylmyrist-oleate (CMO). The latter is obtained from sperm whales and is thought to suppress inflammation and lubricate joints.

For acute episodes of inflammation, Indian ginger (*Zingiber offinalis*) is helpful, as is the German product, Wobenzyme, which is made from a variety of enzymes, including papain, bromelain, trypsin and pancreatin. Apart from its use for arthritis, Wobenzyme is used for sports injuries and muscular strains. Enzymes should always be taken on an empty stomach, together with water or juice.

Rheumatoid arthritis

This is an auto-immune condition, which is not specifically a disease of ageing. Here again, diet is important. Studies have shown that acute symptoms usually resolve when the sufferer is put on a vegan diet, which means eliminating meat, dairy, eggs and other animal products. The African potato (*Hypoxis rooperi*), which contains sterols and sterolins, has also shown considerable success in alleviating the symptoms of rheumatoid arthritis.

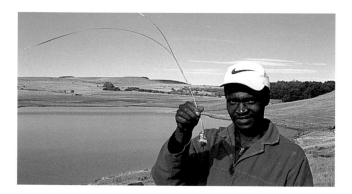

Gout

Gout sufferers may benefit from the Swiss remedy developed by world-renowned naturopath Dr Vogel. This consists of grating raw potato, straining the juice, and drinking about 100ml (3½ fl oz) every morning. Gout may be precipitated by fasting: a fast lasting longer than two days will raise uric acid levels, possibly prompting an attack.

RAW POTATO JUICE

1. Grate a potato or place in a juicer.
2. Strain and combine with an equal amount of carrot juice or water.
3. Drink immediately; do not allow to stand.

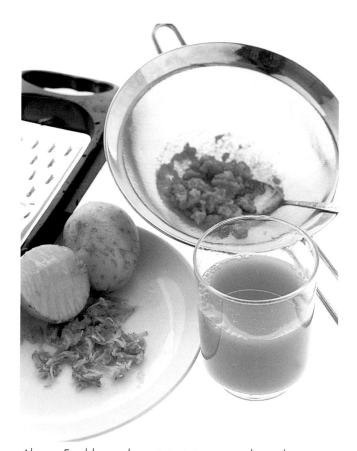

Above: Freshly made potato juice can relieve the painful symptoms of gout.
Left: The African potato has been successful in treating the symptoms of rheumatoid arthritis.

HERBS FOR YOUTHFUL AGEING

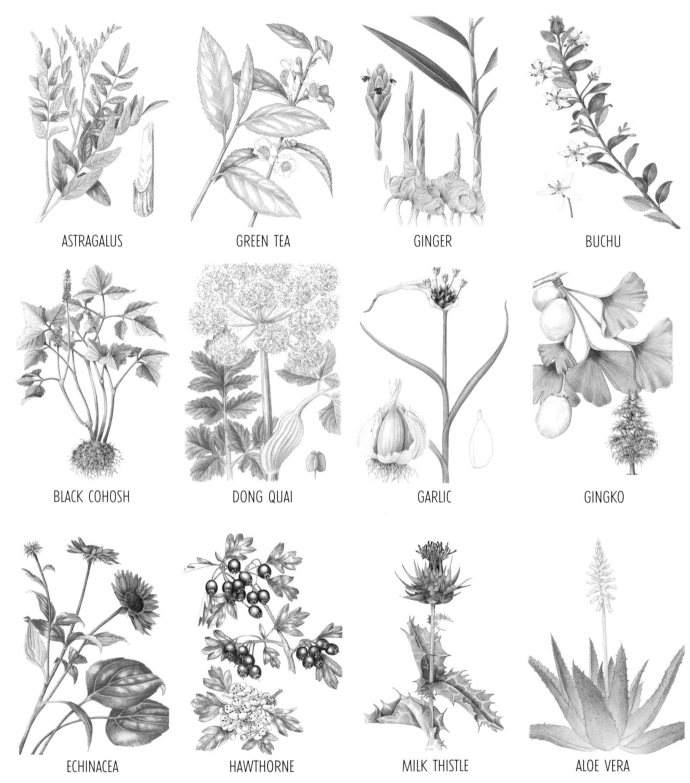

ASTRAGALUS   GREEN TEA   GINGER   BUCHU

BLACK COHOSH   DONG QUAI   GARLIC   GINGKO

ECHINACEA   HAWTHORNE   MILK THISTLE   ALOE VERA

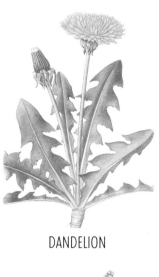

DANDELION

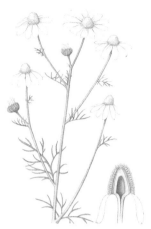

CHAMOMILE

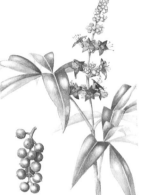
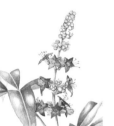

CHASTE TREE

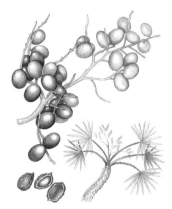

SAW PALMETTO

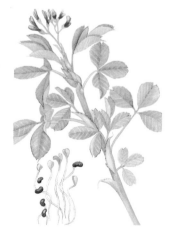

ALFALFA

ROOIBOS / RED BUSH

ORIENTAL AND AFRICAN ANTI-AGEING HERBS

1. *Rehmannia (di huong)* is used by the Chinese as an ingredient in their longevity formulas. It contains plant sterols.

2. *He shou wu* is another Chinese anti-ageing herb and tonic taken by millions of people throughout the East for its rejuvenating properties.

3. *Withania (Ashwaganda)*, known as Indian ginseng, is an Ayurvedic adaptogen used to treat stress and improve male sexual functioning.

4. *Astralagus (huong qi)* is another adaptogen that is used to improve quality of life.

5. *Amrit Kalash* is a potent antioxidant commonly prescribed by Ayurvedic doctors for its rejuvenating properties.

6. *Centella asiatica* promotes scar maturity by stimulating production of Type 1 collagen. It is available as a cream and may be helpful after cosmetic surgery

7. *Sutherlandia*, or the 'cancer bush', is an African medicinal plant known for its use as a multipurpose adaptogenic tonic. Its main function is to boost the immune system.

8. *African potato (Hypoxis rooperi)* has been used by traditional African healers for centuries. Recent research, though not conclusive, seems to suggest immune boosting properties. It also contains plant sterols, which have a beneficial effect on prostatic hypertrophy.

HIGH BLOOD PRESSURE

Lifestyle changes are of primary importance to anyone suffering from high blood pressure. Diet, weight reduction, exercise and stress management often bring blood pressure back to normal. Studies conducted on Seventh Day Adventists in the United States have shown that vegetarians have a 25–30 per cent reduction in the incidence of heart disease, high blood pressure and stroke. Alcohol is another culprit in high blood pressure and stroke. Simply lowering your alcohol intake can bring blood pressure down within normal limits.

Supplements to lower blood pressure:

1. Magnesium relaxes blood vessels. Magnesium citrate, aspartate or orotate are better absorbed than magnesium oxide or chloride. Increase your intake of magnesium-rich foods as well, including leafy green vegetables and whole grains. Research has shown that up to 80 per cent of Western populations are marginally deficient, largely due to the depleted soil in which our vegetables are grown. Certain drugs can cause a deficiency of magnesium, including some diuretics (prescribed for high blood pressure), antibiotics, cortisone, laxatives and alcohol. Magnesium should be taken with meals in doses of 300–400mg, as part of a total multivitamin programme.
2. Vitamin E (tocotrienol) can be taken, 400 units daily.
3. Garlic lowers cholesterol and helps to lower blood pressure.
4. Hawthornberry (*Crataegus*) is a good source of flavonoids, lowering blood pressure and acting as a heart 'tonic'.

Supplements to prevent heart disease and stroke:

1. Resveratrol is a strong antioxidant that protects the heart.
2. Co-enzyme Q10, also known as ubiquinone, is commonly deficient in people with heart disease. Its main benefit lies in strengthening the heart muscle after a heart attack or surgery. As it is fat soluble, take 50mg daily with a meal containing some fat.
3. Carnitine, an amino acid, is essential in the transport of fatty acids into cells. If the heart does not have a good oxygen supply, carnitine levels drop. Supplementation allows the heart muscle to use its reduced oxygen supply more efficiently. Carnitine should be taken together with magnesium. (Note: carnitine should not be confused with acetyl-l-carnitine, which is used as a brain nutrient, or carnosine, which is used as an antioxidant for eye health.)
4. A raised homocysteine level is an independent risk factor for heart disease, and must therefore be treated when it is detected in your baseline blood tests. Homocysteine plays a major role in laying down fatty plaque inside arteries. It can be controlled easily by taking vitamins B6, B12 and folate.
5. Eat more fish. Omega-3 essential fatty acids (EFAs) can be found in herrings, pilchards, salmon and sardines, or as supplements in fish oil capsules. Flaxseed (also known as linseed) is another omega-3 EFA, with the benefit of lowering 'bad' cholesterol and triglycerides in the blood.

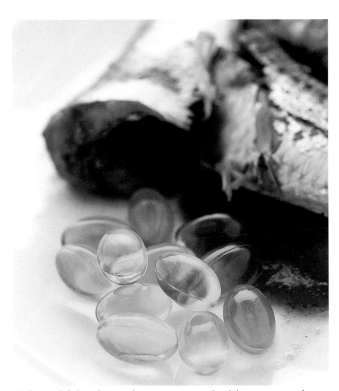

Fish and fish oil supplements are valuable sources of omega-3 fatty acids, which protect against heart disease.

6. Vegetarians may be at risk of developing increased homocysteine levels if they have a low vitamin B12 intake.
7. Niacin, or vitamin B3, lowers blood cholesterol and reduces the formation of blood clots. As a result of minor side effects, such as facial flushing, niacin has been underutilized but remains an alternative to cholesterol-lowering statin drugs.
8. Vitamin E should be used as a blood 'thinner' to prevent clots and thrombosis. It helps to lower the risk of heart attack and stroke.

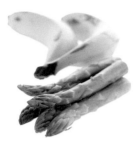

Prebiotic food

DIGESTIVE PROBLEMS

We have already discussed the importance of digestion and the fact that gastric juices and digestive enzymes may decrease as you age (*see* pages 33–34). Absorption is diminished and you may develop a leaky gut. As a result, most people will benefit from digestive aids and supplements to keep the gut milieu well balanced and healthy.

Supplements:
1. For low gastric acid, try one or two teaspoonfuls of apple cider vinegar in 200ml water, taken with meals.
2. Herbal bitters – for example, Schweden bitters, which contains 20 different herbs – stimulate digestion. Take 5ml in a little water.
3. Digestive enzymes aid digestion, but take one without betaine hydrochloride if you suffer from heartburn.
4. A colon-cleansing formula or psyllium husks will assist with constipation and clean out old faecal material.
5. Probiotics – acidophilus and lactobacilli – promote healthy gut bacteria. Make sure that the organisms are viable (alive), and store them in the fridge. To avoid travellers' digestive upsets, or 'Delhi belly', it may be a good idea to take an acidophilus supplement with you when you travel.
6. Eat garlic regularly.
7. To support the liver you could take the herbs milk thistle (*Silybum*), artichoke (*Cynara*) or even dandelion (*Taraxacum*).

8. To enhance the activity of probiotics eat foods rich in fructo-oligosaccharide (FOS), such as asparagus and bananas, which are known as prebiotics.
9. Rooibos tea and chamomile tea are relaxing and antispasmodic. In addition, rooibos tea has antioxidant properties.
10. Ginger tea is beneficial for nausea and indigestion. Infuse two or three slices of fresh ginger in hot water and add a little honey to taste.

There are many arguments for and against the practice of colonic irrigation or colon hydrotherapy. Medical specialists warn against the possibility of perforating the colon, as well as washing out the good bacteria along with the bad, resulting in diarrhoea. However, there is some merit if you are suffering from chronic constipation or overgrowth of bad bacteria, such as Candida. Choose a well-trained therapist in a clinic that has state-of-the-art equipment. After treatment, friendly bacteria or probiotics should be given.

CLEANSING PSYLLIUM SHAKE

1. Add two teaspoons of psyllium husk powder to a glass of water.
2. Stir briskly.
3. Drink immediately (the mixture gels quickly) and follow this with another glass of water, or half water/half juice.
4. Drink your shake early in the morning – at least one hour before breakfast, which ideally should consist only of fruit.

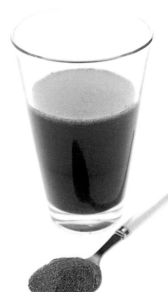

BLOOD SUGAR CONTROL

Elevated or fluctuating blood sugar, known as dysglycemia, is a serious risk factor in premature ageing. In its most severe form we have maturity onset or Type 2 diabetes. We also have Syndrome X or metabolic syndrome, the hallmarks of which include insulin resistance, abdominal adiposity, high blood pressure and an increased risk of heart disease. In both these disorders, and in the normal course of ageing, there is protein glycation or 'AGEs'. This is when blood sugar combines with protein to form a sticky compound, resulting in accelerated ageing of all body parts.

To prevent blood sugar fluctuations, diet is the firstline defence. The Glycaemic Index (GI) diet is one that chooses foods with a low glycaemic index. It is based on the fact that not all carbohydrates are equal. Some increase blood sugar levels more than others and these are the ones rated as having a high GI. The glycaemic index is rated from 1 to 100. Foods with a low GI include fruit, vegetables, legumes and whole grains. The undesirable foods with a high GI include sugar and refined carbohydrates, cakes, cookies, desserts and white bread. Sugar rates as 100 on the GI scale, whereas fruit and vegetables rate at approximately 30. In addition to choosing low GI foods, make sure that you include adequate protein in your diet. All this fits in with the recommendations for healthy eating.

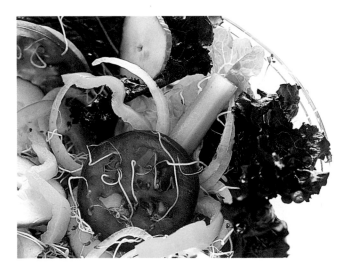

Supplements:
1. For sugar cravings and improved glucose tolerance, take 200 micrograms chromium or Brewer's yeast.
2. Take 300mg magnesium and 15–20mg zinc at night, together with 500mg vitamin C and 400 units of vitamin E in the morning.
3. Take alpha lipoic acid (ALA), 50–100mg daily.

LOW GLYCAEMIC INDEX (< 55)
Yoghurt, low-fat milk
Wholewheat bread
High-fibre bran cereal, oats, muesli
Basmati rice, pasta, noodles
Soya products
Lentils, chick peas, beans, baked beans
All deciduous and citrus fruits
Corn on the cob, sweet potato
Leafy green vegetables

INTERMEDIATE GLYCAEMIC INDEX (55–70)
Ryebread, pita bread, Ryvita
White rice, couscous
Tropical fruit, bananas, mango, pineapple
Raisins and sultanas
Bran muffins
Bran flakes, instant oats

HIGH GLYCAEMIC INDEX (> 70)
White bread, rice cakes, bagels, croissants
Puffed wheat, corn flakes, rice crispies
Watermelon
Carrots and carrot juice
Potatoes (boiled or baked), chips
Pumpkin, butternut, hubbard squash
Biscuits, sweets, cakes, desserts
White pasta
Honey, sugar

OSTEOPOROSIS

Nowadays, people are living longer, so it is essential to look after our bones and joints. Osteoporosis is today recognized as a major health concern in the Western world. In the United States alone it affects 28 million people, and one out of two women older than 50 will sustain an osteoporosis-related fracture during her lifetime. Men may also develop osteoporosis. Their risk factors include hypogonadism or low levels of male hormones. In the United States, about 1.5 million men over the age of 65 have osteoporosis. The lifetime risk of fracture for men is 25 per cent at the age of 60.

Supplementation is essential for people who have been found to have a low bone mineral density on baseline testing, but it is also advisable for all adults over the age of 40. Risk factors for both men and women include alcohol, medications such as steroids, dieting, eating disorders, smoking and a family history of osteoporosis.

Supplements:
1. Magnesium is essential: about 300–400mg daily. Take together with 500–800mg calcium in a ratio of 2:3.
2. 5–10mg boron may be added to the calcium-magnesium combination.
3. Avoid carbonated drinks and excessive meat consumption. Both contain phosphates that combine with calcium, which is then excreted and lost – promoting bone loss.
4. One or two teaspoonsful of apple cider vinegar and honey in warm water helps to assimilate calcium. It also combats low stomach acidity. Gastric acid declines with age, impairing calcium absorption.
5. Soy isoflavones found in soya products have been shown to increase bone mineral density.

WANING HORMONES
Growth hormone

Growth hormone (HGH), known as the 'master hormone of youth', is produced by the pituitary gland in a pulsing motion. If too little is produced it can promote dwarfism; too much creates giantism. As we age, HGH production declines: by the age of 65, 35 per cent of us are deficient in HGH. Does a low level of HGH shorten lifespan? It seems not. But studies of HGH replacement in older people have shown that it improves quality of life, wellbeing and sexual potency. It also improves memory and skin elasticity, increases muscle mass without exercise, and promotes fat loss without dieting. All of these benefits are most attractive to a normally ageing individual.

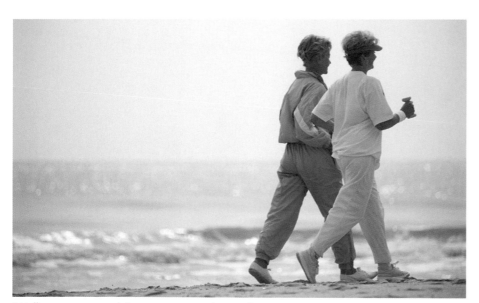

Walking is essential for maintaining bone density to prevent osteoporosis.

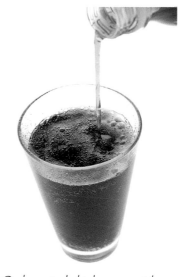

Carbonated drinks are a risk factor for osteoporosis.

THE MULTIHORMONE ORCHESTRA

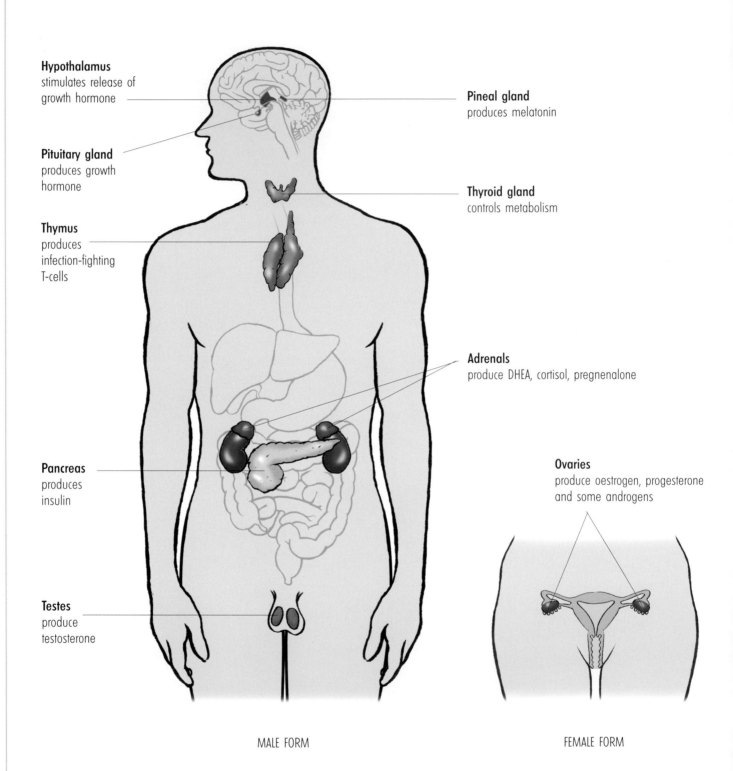

Hypothalamus
stimulates release of
growth hormone

Pituitary gland
produces growth
hormone

Thymus
produces
infection-fighting
T-cells

Pancreas
produces
insulin

Testes
produce
testosterone

Pineal gland
produces melatonin

Thyroid gland
controls metabolism

Adrenals
produce DHEA, cortisol, pregnenalone

Ovaries
produce oestrogen, progesterone
and some androgens

MALE FORM

FEMALE FORM

HGH is usually administered by injection, implant or sublingual (under the tongue) spray. However, there are significant side effects. The most common include fluid retention, joint pains and carpal tunnel syndrome. High blood pressure, diabetes, gynaeco-mastia – breast growth in men – and even cancer have also been implicated.

Is there any way to stimulate the pituitary gland to release HGH, using natural methods? The answer is yes – by exercise that includes both aerobic and resistance training. HGH is also released during fasting, which is another good reason to have a detox day once a week. A further option would be to supplement with secretagogues, which offer an attractive alternative to HGH supplementation as an anti-ageing treatment.

Secretagogues

Secretagogues are natural amino acids, which are the building blocks of protein. They stimulate the pituitary gland to release HGH. The main secreta-gogues are arginine, ornithine, glutamine and lysine. As a supplement, they are taken in combination.

Athletes use them as part of their nutritional support regime. Benefits include improved muscle building, increased fat burning, better immunity, higher energy levels and improved sexual performance in men. Arginine has the interesting property of stimulating the production of nitric oxide in the body, one of the effects of which is sexual arousal. It has therefore been called 'poor man's Viagra'.

'Cocktails' of secreta-gogues should be taken on an empty stomach, five days a week, with one month off every three months so as not to interfere with the body's natural production.

Pregnenalone

This prehormone is produced in the body from cholesterol, and is the base hormone of the steroid hormones DHEA, progesterone, testosterone and oestrogen. It appears to block the effect of the stress hormone, cortisol. As an anti-ageing supplement it is reportedly safe and has the benefits of improving memory and mood, and possibly even bone mineral density. It is also useful for the perimenopause – that is, the period between the ages of 45 to 50, immediately preceding the menopause. We are still in the early stages of pregnenalone research and do not know about its long-term effects when used as hormone replacement therapy.

As a supplement it is manufactured from the wild yam, and the recommended daily dose is 3–10mg.

DHEA

Dehydroepiandrosterone (DHEA), produced by the adrenal glands, is further down on the steroid cascade. Levels decline with age so that by age 65 your body's levels have reduced to 20 per cent of what they were when you were 30. You can have your level checked in your baseline blood tests. There are also saliva tests for DHEA levels.

Many anti-ageing benefits have been claimed, including improved immunity and reduced risk of age-related diseases. DHEA also acts as a buffer against the stress hormone, cortisol, so is beneficial in helping to cope with anxiety and tension. The French researcher, Professor Etienne-Emile Baulieu, has found that DHEA supplementation helps to improve older women's libido, skin texture and bone density. Although DHEA appears to be safe, its long-term effects are unknown.

DHEA is converted into testosterone and oestrogen and should not be taken by anyone with a history of prostate, breast or ovarian cancer. If you decide to supplement with DHEA, start with a small dose of 5–15mg for women, and 10–25mg for men on alternate days. Have your DHEA blood levels checked every six months. A natural way to increase your DHEA levels is by exercise.

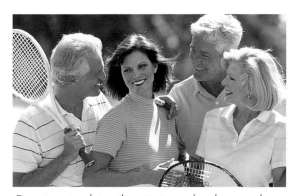

Exercise stimulates the pituitary gland to produce human growth hormone (HGH), and increases DHEA levels.

Multihormone replacement

Anti-ageing physicians may prescribe a combined hormone replacement programme to recreate the hormone profile of youth. For men, this may include growth hormone or HGH secretagogues, melatonin, DHEA and testosterone. For women, oestrogen, progesterone, DHEA or pregnenolone, thyroid and melatonin could be used. Oestrogen may not prevent heart disease, as was thought previously, but it does plump out skin, adding moisture and collagen, as well as controlling urogenital ageing. Women taking oestrogen replacement have a 50 per cent reduced risk of Alzheimer's disease. Oestrogen also protects bone and prevents osteoporosis, but there is a small increase in the risk of breast cancer.

If you decide to take oestrogen replacement, ask your doctor for 'bio-identical' oestrogen. If progesterone is required, use micronized oral progesterone rather than synthetic 'progestins'.

With all the doubts about the safety of oestrogen therapy, many women prefer to use alternative herbal supplements known as plant or phyto-oestrogens, which are quite safe. These include black cohosh, red clover and soy isoflavones. Red clover contains four isoflavones, compared to two in soy products. Although red clover has not been extensively researched, it has a modest effect on hot flushes and is reported to increase bone mineral density.

Isoflavones may protect the heart due to their ability to cause vasodilation or widening of the blood vessels. Soy isoflavones also improve bone density. As a result, soy products and foods containing phyto-oestrogens, such as chickpeas and lentils, would seem to be beneficial additions to every woman's diet. They

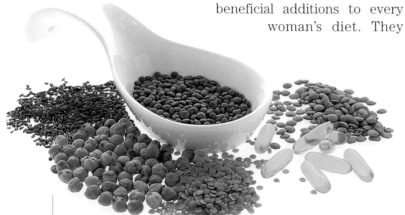

help to protect against breast cancer and should be combined with daily intake of linseed or flaxseed oil.

In future we may even be prescribed a single transdermal patch that contains an individualized multihormone cocktail.

The perimenopause

This includes women in the age group of 40 to 50. It is the time when a woman's body gets ready for the menopause, and its symptoms are similar. Menstruation becomes irregular, and hot flushes and night sweats may occur. Some women experience depression, fatigue and mood swings associated with hormonal changes. Doctors may prescribe oestrogens, but herbal remedies are often helpful. Dong quai (*Angelica sinensis*), chasteberry (*Vitex agnus castus*), black cohosh and red clover are phyto-oestrogens that can be effective in alleviating hormone-related symptoms. Soy isoflavones and flaxseed should be included.

MULTIHORMONE REPLACEMENT FOR MEN	MULTIHORMONE REPLACEMENT FOR WOMEN
Growth hormone or secretagogues Melatonin Testosterone DHEA	Bio-identical oestrogen (with or without progesterone) OR soy isoflavones, red clover, black cohosh Thyroid Melatonin DHEA or pregnenolone

Male menopause (andropause)

Ageing in men is accompanied by a gradual but progressive reduction in testosterone levels, growth hormone, DHEA and melatonin. The testosterone deficiency syndrome that usually occurs in a man's late fifties – but may occur as early as the mid-forties or as late as in the sixties – is called the andropause. The term derives from the fact that testosterone is an androgen steroid hormone. The andropause should not be confused with the mid-life crisis, which is essentially emotional in origin and usually starts in the mid-forties.

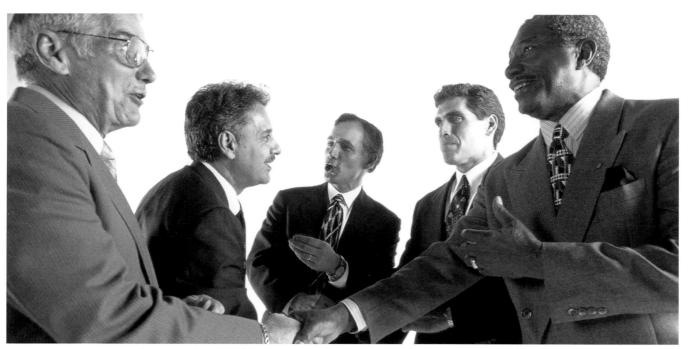

Business executives may become depressed on retirement; this may be confused with or coincide with testosterone deficiency.

Do men need testosterone replacement therapy? What are the symptoms of waning hormone levels? The most common are depression, irritability, low energy, decreased vigour, and decreased muscle mass and strength. From middle age a man may develop erectile dysfunction, impaired libido and fat accumulation around the waist. Some degree of erectile dysfunction is found in 52 per cent of men over 40. Smokers are twice as likely to develop erectile dysfunction, as are men with a body mass index (BMI) of more than 28, which is classified as obese. Men with a high cholesterol or low DHEA levels are also at risk.

The problem with initial diagnosis is that when men retire at the age of 60 or 65, they may become depressed and exhibit many of the symptoms of testosterone deficiency. A man who has the symptoms described above should have his hormone levels checked, remembering that testosterone levels can drop in young men as well. A study conducted in Italy on healthy young men in their twenties showed that eating substantial amounts of liquorice inhibited testosterone production.

Testosterone replacement may be by injection, transdermal gel or skin patch. Prostate health must be checked carefully, and prostate-specific antigen blood tests should be performed annually, together with digital examination.

There are numerous benefits of testosterone replacement therapy.
- Improved body composition with increased lean and reduced fat
- Increased muscle strength
- Improved bone mineral density
- Increased libido and sexual functioning
- Improved memory and mood

However, there are also some risks.
- Possible increase in prostatic hypertrophy (enlargement)
- Possible hastening of prostate cancer
- Fluid retention
- Breast development

Physical exercise is still the safest approach to anti-ageing in males. A natural way to increase testosterone production, as well as that of your growth hormone, DHEA and melatonin levels, is to practise 'dinner cancelling' – which means eating very little or nothing for the evening meal.

Female androgen deficiency syndrome

Androgens (testosterone) have traditionally been thought to be male hormones. However, women produce them throughout their lives. Both testosterone and DHEA are produced by the adrenal glands and both of these prehormones decline with age so that women in their forties have half the level of circulating testosterone of women in their twenties.

What are the symptoms of androgen deficiency in women? Suggested symptoms include low libido, decreased sexual enjoyment, loss of muscle tone and low energy levels. These symptoms can also be attributed to other causes – for example, depression. Women's health clinicians have found that supplementing with testosterone in women who have had their ovaries removed results in significant improvements in their mood and sexual functioning.

The risks and side effects of treatment are acne and facial hair, whereas the benefits include an increase in lean tissue, muscle strength and bone mineral density.

Researchers have concluded that androgen therapy may be useful for women who have lowered mood and sexual dysfunction, if other causes are excluded. However, there is still inadequate data to recommend its use routinely.

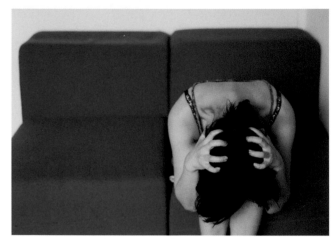

Depression can be a sign of androgen deficiency.

THE AGEING BODY	WHAT HAPPENS	WHAT HELPS
Heart and vascular system	Blood pressure increases Heart pump becomes less efficient Fatty plaque buildup in blood vessels Poor circulation Raised homocysteine levels	Magnesium, vitamin E, omega-3 essential fatty acids Hawthornberry, co-enzyme Q10, carnitine Niacin (B3), garlic, resveratrol Ginkgo Vitamin B6, B12, folate
Brain and nervous system	Memory loss Insomnia Depression Anxiety	ALA, vitamin E and C, Amrit Kalash, pregnenolone Melatonin Sceletium, magnesium, vitamin B complex Valerian, magnesium, chamomile
Bones and joints	Loss of bone mineral density Osteoporosis Cartilage deterioration Osteoarthritis Rheumatoid arthritis Gout	Calcium, magnesium, boron Soy isoflavones Glucosamine, chondroitin, MSM Pycnogenol, vitamin E, fish oil African potato, Indian ginger, Wobenzyme Potato juice, buchu tea
Muscles and body shape	Loss of lean tissue Increase in fat Body composition changes Increased abdominal fat	HGH secretagogues Colostrum L-carnitine Exercise

THE AGEING BODY	WHAT HAPPENS	WHAT HELPS
Immune system	Declining immune function and susceptibility to infections and disease	Sutherlandia, astragalus, shiitake, echinacea, sterols and sterolins, African potato, Amrit Kalash, zinc, vitamin C, chlorella
Adrenal glands	Cortisol stress hormone increases	DHEA, magnesium, eleutherococcus (Siberian ginseng), pregnenolone
Thyroid	Subclinical hypothyroidism common in women	Kelp, zinc, thyroxine
Digestive tract	Low stomach acid Fewer digestive enzymes Absorption declines Liver detox impaired Constipation Nausea, indigestion Spastic colon	Cider vinegar, herbal bitters Digestive enzymes Probiotics, garlic Milk thistle, dandelion, artichoke, beetroot Psyllium husks, acidophilus, fructo-oligosaccharides Ginger tea, slippery elm Rooibos tea, chamomile, aloe vera
Skin	Dermis becomes thinner Photo-ageing and pigmentation Wrinkles	ALA, vitamin A, vitamin C, MSM *Kigelia africana* cream Gotu kola (*Centella asiatica*) after cosmetic surgery
Eyes	Dry eyes Cataract Macular degeneration Glaucoma	Omega-3 essential fatty acids Euphrasia (eyebright) Lutein and zeaxanthin (carotenoids) Bilberry, l-carnosine
Ears	Hearing loss Tinnitus	Antioxidants Ginkgo biloba
Hair	Thinning, hair loss	Kelp, biotin, inositol, choline, zinc, MSM, vitamin B
Teeth	Gum disease	Propolis, co-enzyme Q10, vitamin C, Rutin
Pancreas	Insulin resistance, poor blood sugar control and Syndrome X	ALA, chromium, vitamin C, magnesium, carnosine, fenugreek, buchu
Kidneys and bladder	Poor bladder control, incontinence	Cranberry
Prostate	Enlargement / hypertrophy	African potato, sterols and sterolins, saw palmetto, zinc, lycopene
Female sex hormones	Menopause	HRT or phyto-oestrogens, black cohosh, soy isoflavones, red clover, DHEA, pregnenalone
Male sex hormones	Andropause	Testosterone replacement therapy, growth hormone or secretagogues, DHEA, melatonin

As we grow older, we have different requirements. Here are a few suggestions for supplements that may be beneficial for each decade.

THIRTIES

30s

You should be at your peak, but start now to prevent loss of lean tissue, maintain healthy bones and prevent degenerative disorders.

SUPPLEMENT	WHAT IT DOES	WHAT ITS GOOD FOR
Multivitamin and mineral combination	Provides cocktail of essential vitamins and minerals	Preventive maintenance
Magnesium	Muscle relaxant, bone builder	Premenstrual syndrome, stress, healthy bones
Antioxidants	Fight free radicals	Environmental pollution

FORTIES

40s

You should be in good health. Metabolism is slowing down, so watch your weight. Men may develop a midlife crisis, while women are approaching the perimenopause. Watch blood pressure and blood sugar levels.

Vitamin E	Antioxidant	Helps circulation, prevents heart disease and stroke
Acidophilus	Probiotics feed the good gut bacteria	Intestinal good health
Eleutherococcus (Siberian ginseng)	Adaptogen, supports the adrenal glands	Stress, fatigue
Valerian, passiflora	Induces relaxation	Anxiety, insomnia
ALA, lipoic acid	Antioxidant	Prevents diabetes and skin ageing, promotes liver detox
Soy isoflavones for women	Natural plant oestrogens	Perimenopause
Omega-3 essential fatty acids	Anti-inflammatory	Reduces risk of arthritis and heart disease, promotes healthy skin

FIFTIES

50s

Focus on reducing your risk for life-threatening diseases such as cancer, heart disease and stroke.

Resveratrol	Potent antioxidant	Anti-cancer, prevents heart disease
Magnesium + calcium + boron combination	Promotes bone health	Osteoporosis
Co-enzyme Q10	Co-worker with vitamins C and E	Heart disease
African potato	Plant sterols and sterolins boost immunity	Prostate health, boosting immune system
Digestive enzymes	Assist food digestion	Intestinal health
Amrit Kalash	Antioxidant	Prevents degenerative diseases

SIXTIES

You should still be vigorous and healthy. Focus on boosting immunity, and preventing degenerative diseases and Alzheimer's disease.

60s

SUPPLEMENT	WHAT IT DOES	WHAT ITS GOOD FOR
Vitamin E	Antioxidant	Heart, blood pressure, circulation, skin, joints
Resveratrol	Antioxidant	Vascular system, anti-cancer
Magnesium + calcium + boron	Promotes bone health	Osteoporosis, arthritis
Melatonin	Antioxidant, anti-ageing, promotes good sleep	Insomnia
Saw palmetto	Controls prostate size	Prostate enlargement
General multivitamin with zinc	Synergistic vitamins and minerals work together	Nutrient cocktail
Digestive enzymes	Assist in food digestion	Intestinal health

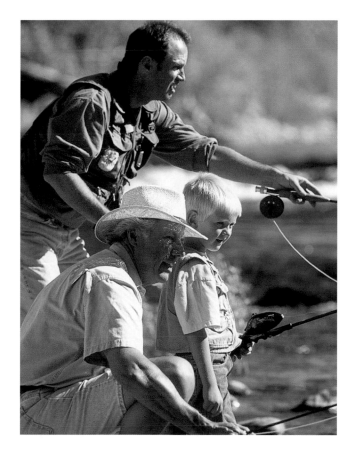

ACTION PLAN

➤ For daily use, choose a multivitamin and mineral combination from a reputable company.

➤ Add to this an antioxidant formula appropriate to your needs.

➤ Supplements suggested for various health problems associated with ageing are helpful for prevention, as well as for alleviation, of current symptoms.

➤ Refer to the seven risk factors for premature ageing (*see* pages 20–29) and ensure that you take preventive action.

➤ Remember that extra vitamins, minerals and herbs are only as good as the diet accompanying them.

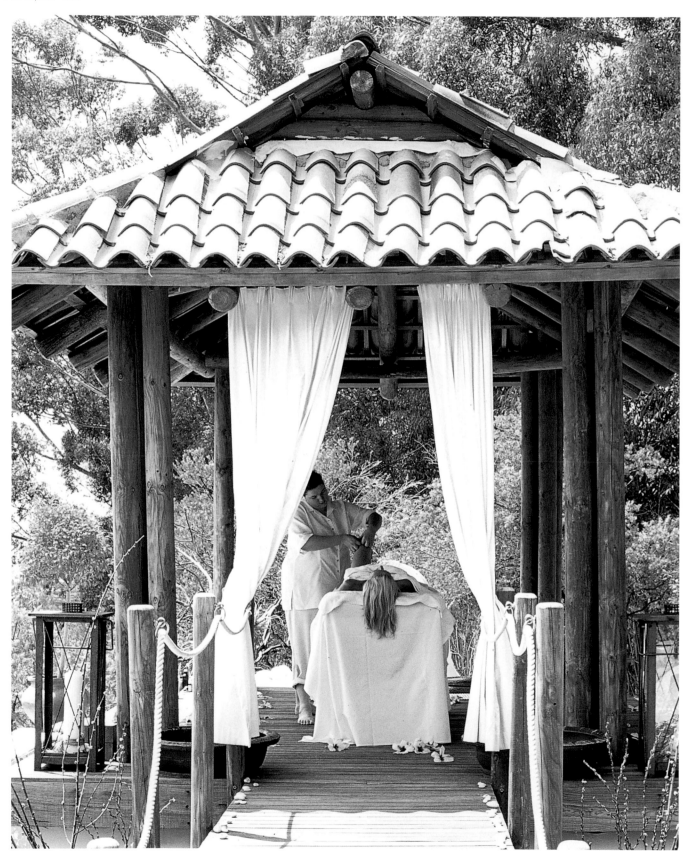

*Massage is an excellent body-mind therapy that improves circulation, drains lymphatics and relaxes muscles.
Endorphins or 'happiness hormones' are released to counteract anxiety, depression and stress-related symptoms.*

SPA THERAPIES

When we think of spa therapies and the spa experience, the word 'blissful' comes to mind. Spa therapies make us feel pampered, relaxed, rejuvenated and energized. We feel healthier, destressed, detoxified and definitely younger. We emerge glowing and remotivated. We decide to really watch our diet, exercise daily and take time out for relaxation.

There has been an enormous explosion in the health and wellness industry in recent years. In developed countries life expectancy has increased and individuals want to stay young for as long as possible. There has been a paradigm shift in medical care. The old medical model still taught at medical schools concentrates on treating disease and symptoms with drugs or surgery. A frustrated public has moved towards self-care and natural therapies. Pharmaceutical drugs are lifesaving for acute illnesses, but at least 70 per cent of illnesses are chronic and can be treated by a change in diet, regular detoxification, appropriate supplementation and exercise. Drugs such as anti-inflammatories, blood pressure pills and tranquillizers are seriously ageing. Apart from anything else, they may contribute to a leaky gut and a toxic liver.

We are living in a very fast-paced society, which results in a tremendous increase in the number of stress-related disorders. Rather than resorting to medications, many people are consulting complementary therapists or taking themselves off to spas, retreats and wellness resorts.

The growth of the spa industry in the United States reflects the international trend: in 1990, there were 1300 spas; in 1999, the number had increased to 6000. Revenues from spas are estimated at US$6 billion,

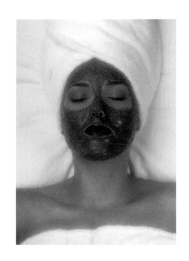

Seaweed facial mask

with 95 million spa visitors annually. Spas are increasingly being added to hotels and resorts, and a new trend is towards medical spas where multidisciplinary teams of doctors work with dieticians, psychologists, and massage and beauty therapists.

THE MIND-BODY CONNECTION

The mind has a profound effect on the body. Each thought is transmitted to every one of our trillion cells, our tissues and our organs. Our thoughts can be ageing or anti-ageing. In his book, *Grow Younger Live Longer*, Deepak Chopra recommends that we use our minds to think ourselves younger. As a well-known guru of alternative medicine, Chopra's approach combines Eastern philosophy and wisdom with Western scientific knowledge.

Our feelings and emotions have a powerful effect on our vital body organs. Of the three most toxic emotions – namely, anxiety, depression and anger – it is anger that seriously damages the heart. When we are stressed, the adrenal glands pour out cortisol, which damages brain cells. In addition, when we are stressed, the immune system shuts down. Killer cells are deactivated and we become vulnerable to invading bacteria, viruses and even cancer cells. Chronic stress promotes insulin resistance, with out-of-control blood sugar. Stress impairs digestion and creates turmoil in the gut.

Excess cortisol is the most ageing and damaging substance in our bodies. Instead of diminishing as we age, it actually increases, so we do not need toxic emotions or stress to aggravate the situation. It is abundantly clear that stress reduction through body-mind therapies is a most effective way of staying youthful and preventing degenerative disease.

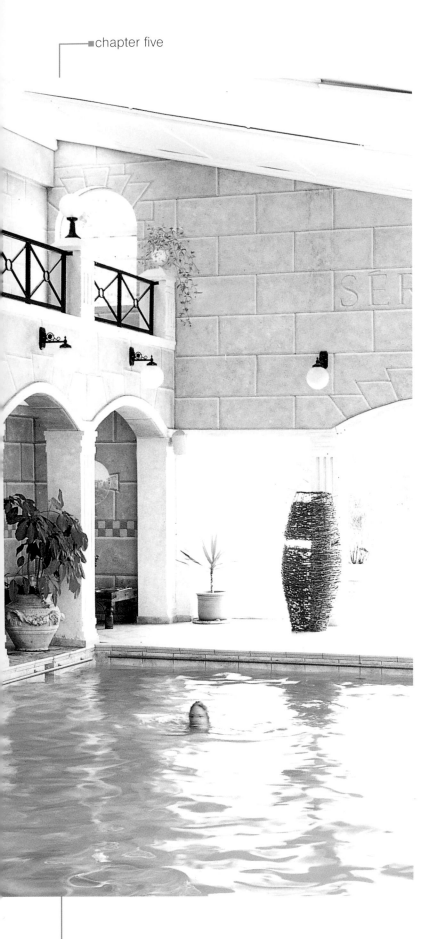

The science of psycho-neuroimmunology has now become mainstream. It has been irrefutably established that there is an inseparable relationship between the mind and the body. For example, studies have been conducted on university students who are known to become prone to colds and flu before examinations. It has been found that stress depresses students' killer cells, which are important white blood cells involved in the immune system and are responsible for protecting the body from invading viruses, bacteria and other organisms.

Successful ageing will be enhanced by the therapies described in this chapter. You do not have to book into a residential spa: you can treat yourself at a day spa, visit your favourite therapist, or even practise some of the therapies in your own home.

Stress is not the only reason why experiencing these therapies is recommended. They are a form of preventive maintenance and should be a part of everyone's daily or weekly routine.

What are the anti-ageing benefits of spa therapies?

1. Cortisol production is slowed down to normal limits.
2. Circulation is improved. Blood flow that carries nutrients and oxygen to tissues is enhanced.
3. Tense muscles are relaxed.
4. Stiff joints are mobilized.
5. The brain is 'unscrambled' and balance is created between right and left sides.
6. Detoxification through the skin, kidneys and liver is improved.
7. Meridians or energy pathways in the body are unblocked.
8. The metabolism is stimulated, which helps to promote weight loss.
9. Beta-endorphins – natural 'happiness' hormones – are released, giving us a feeling of wellbeing.
10. The lymphatic system is activated.

Left: Swimming promotes fitness and is an excellent way to reduce stress. High levels of the stress hormone, cortisol, damage both the immune system and brain cells.

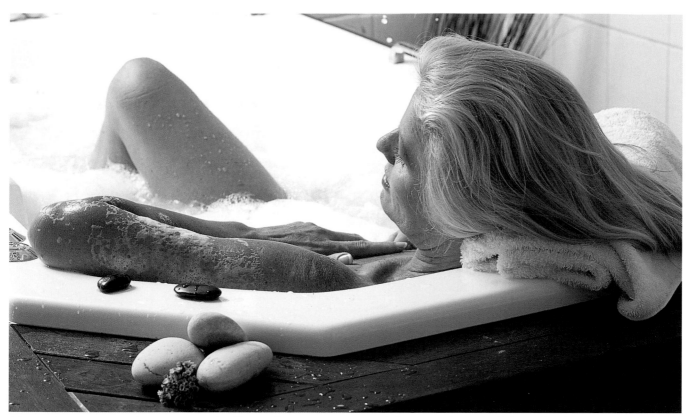

Thermal spa waters relieve pain and stiffness. They may contain sulphur or radon, which have healing properties that have been shown to help relieve many musculoskeletal illnesses.

HYDROTHERAPY

From earliest times, water has been recognized to have therapeutic properties. The word 'hydro', meaning water, was formerly attached to places of healing. The Greek physician, Galen, who lived in AD200 had hydrotherapy pools fed by 'sacred springs' in his temple of Aesclepius near Pergamon in Turkey. Wherever they colonized, the Romans, too, built bathhouses, which were forerunners of today's day spas. Beautifully designed and decorated, they incorporated steam rooms, hot and cold bathing pools, and massage and aromatherapy rooms. For the Romans, spending time each day at a day spa was a form of preventive maintenance and not just a hedonistic feel-good experience.

In fact, ritual bathing for the purpose of cleansing the mind and body has been a part of Indian, Christian and African cultures since time immemorial. During the 18th and 19th centuries it became fashionable to 'take the waters' at places such as

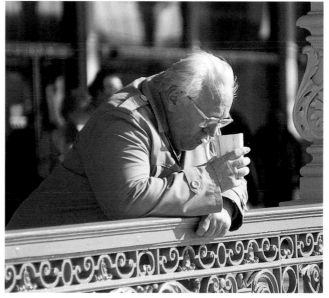

'Taking the waters' is a popular health regimen in Europe, where the mineral spa waters benefit chronic ailments such as arthritis and digestive disorders.

Karlsbad (Karlovy Vary), Vichy and Baden-Baden. The British King Edward VII travelled to Bad Homberg for his annual cleanse and detox, where he was followed by the King of Siam, Czar Nicholas II of Russia and several kings from central Europe.

More recently, mineral water therapy or thermal 'cures' have become popular at spas in Germany, France, Italy, Austria, the Czech Republic, Slovakia and Hungary. The practice of both drinking and bathing in natural mineral water was – and still is – recognized as having therapeutic benefits.

In contemporary times many scientific papers have been published, and the German-based International Society of Medical Hydrology meets regularly to discuss the applications of water therapies. However, hydrotherapy has largely been neglected in other countries as a serious means of health maintenance and treatment of chronic ailments such as arthritis and musculoskeletal disorders.

What are hydrotherapy's effects?

One of the basic laws of hydrotherapy is that of action and reaction. Application of any form of heat to the skin forces blood to the surface, whereas application of cold water has the initial effect of driving blood away from the surface. The secondary and lasting effect is that of warmth, since by the law of action and reaction the blood must circulate back to the vessels and tissues from which it was expelled. This law can best be seen at work in the three basic hydrotherapy baths – hot, cold and alternating hot and cold.

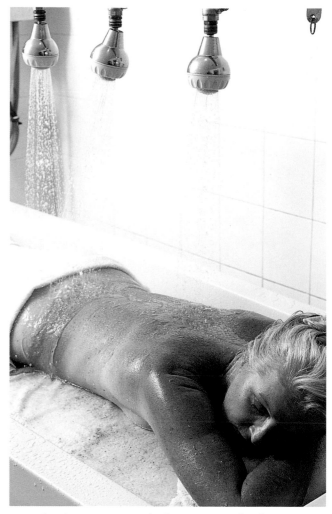

A Vichy shower uses multiple jets to apply alternating hot and cold water. This stimulates the circulation and boosts the immune system.

APPLICATION OF COLD WATER	APPLICATION OF HOT WATER
Lowers heart rate	Increases heart rate
First increases then lowers blood pressure	Increases then lowers blood pressure
Skin: increases tone	Skin: sweating and fluid loss
Increases metabolic rate	
Increases muscle tone	Muscle relaxation
Stimulating effect	Enervating effect
	Causes diuresis, with increased urine output

What are its benefits?

1. It relieves muscular tension, helping to reduce pain and stiffness.
2. Jets and hoses serve to stimulate blood circulation and lymph drainage.
3. Alternating warm and cold applications stimulate the immune system. Incidence of colds and flu is dramatically reduced with continued use.
4. It releases endorphins, a process that creates a general feeling of wellbeing.
5. Combined with diet and exercise, the increase in metabolic rate promotes weight loss.

6. Mineral or thermal waters have specific properties – for example, sulphur-rich baths are excellent for arthritis and skin disorders, while radon baths have a dramatic effect on rheumatoid and other forms of arthritis.

7. Immersion in water results in increased urine output, or diuresis, and helps to treat fluid retention. At Bath Spa in the United Kingdom a research project was conducted on subjects immersed in water maintained at 35°C (95°F) for two hours. The result was a significant increase in urine output and an average weight loss of 5kg (11 lb). This validates the centuries-old practice of spa treatment for many disease conditions. An interesting finding was that there was no difference between the use of thermal water and tap water.

8. Hydrotherapy is an excellent means of treating stress. A soak in a warm bath, perhaps with added aromatherapy essences, will lower cortisol levels.

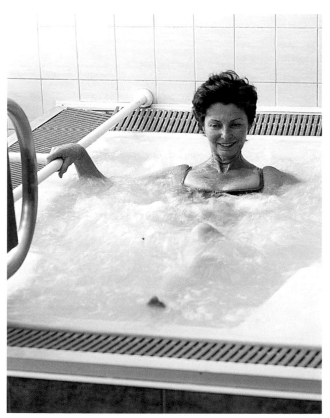

The hydropool applies jet massage to specific problem areas such as a stiff neck or tense shoulders.

What forms are found at modern spas?

1. *Jacuzzis*: these can be either with or without underwater massage hoses.

2. *Alternating hot and cold baths:* the Kneipp method, initially developed by German Catholic priest Father Sebastian Kneipp, has a stimulating effect on the circulation and the immune system. Kneipp therapies include changing foot and arm baths, water treading in outdoor pools, hosing and affusion, which is a slow stream of water. Changing footbaths may be beneficial for circulatory diseases, tired or 'heavy' legs, and insomnia. Hosing is good for varicose veins.

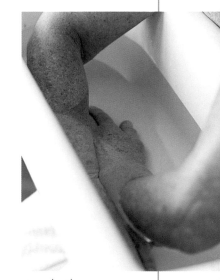

Arm bath

3. *Hydropools*: these are much larger than jacuzzis and have powerful jets on the side walls that can be applied to the back or other parts of the body. These pools have shallow areas where you can lie on a shelf with multiple underwater jets spraying upwards to give the sensation of floating on water.

4. *Liquid sound:* this is a truly feel-good experience. Bathing in a saline pool is accompanied by underwater music. There may be changing soft-coloured lights overhead so that you are bathing in light and sound.

5. *Flotation tanks:* this is primarily a means of stress reduction, known as 'restricted environmental stimulation therapy' or REST. Inside a capsule, you float in shallow saline water – rather like floating in the Dead Sea – in total darkness and silence. In addition, there may be subliminal stress-reducing tapes or music.

6. *Vichy showers:* here you lie on a bed with an overhead row of multiple showers spraying your body from top to toe. Temperature can be varied and this is a good way to stimulate circulation.

7. *Scottish douche:* the therapist, holding a hose, aims a powerful jet of – usually cold – water at the

subject. Moving the hose up and down the body has a powerful stimulating effect on the circulation.

8. *Sitz baths:* you sit in a hipbath so your lower abdomen is covered in warm water. After three minutes you move to a second hipbath containing cold water, where you sit for a minute. This process is repeated three times. The beneficial effect on the pelvic organs is useful for prostatic hypertrophy (enlargement), haemorrhoids and menstrual problems.

Can you practise hydrotherapy at home?

Yes, all you require is a shower, either overhead or a hand shower, and hot and cold water. Changing foot-baths according to the Kneipp method can be successful using two plastic buckets. You can even use a hosepipe in the garden to rev up your circulation.

One of the most beneficial practices everyone should implement as a daily routine is to take a shower. Start off with warm water, and then turn on

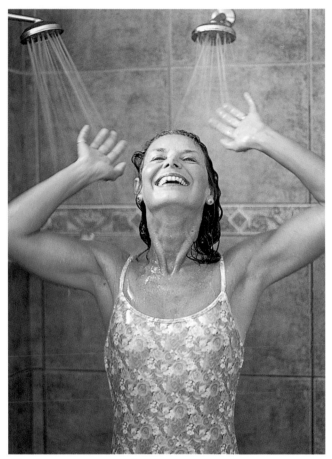

Showering is an excellent way to generate negative ions and stimulate the immune system.

the cold water for at least one minute. You will feel invigorated and will probably never catch a cold again. The secret is to apply cold water to a thoroughly warmed body but never to apply cold water to a cold body.

SKIN BRUSHING

Before experiencing body treatments such as seaweed wraps, it is essential to exfoliate the skin. In fact, daily dry skin brushing should be a part of everyone's health regime.

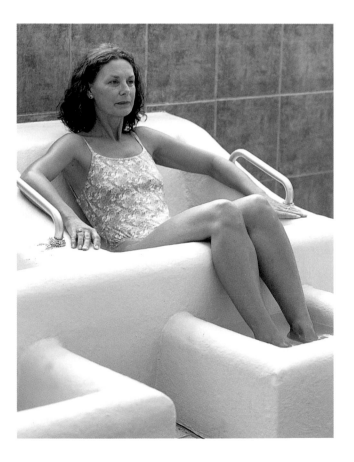

Left: The sitz bath targets pelvic organs. Alternating hot and cold immersions benefit prostate health in men and menstrual disorders in women.

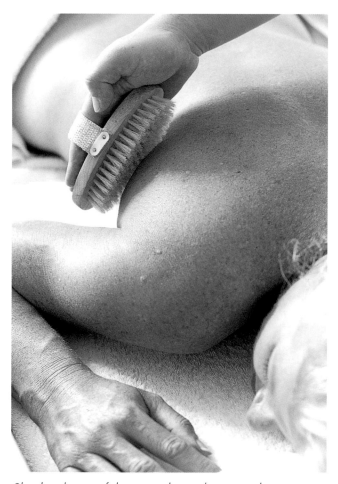

Skin brushing exfoliates and stimulates circulation.

What are the benefits?

- The most important is the shedding of dead skin cells. As we age, the superficial skin layer becomes thinner and more delicate, so a soft brush is preferable to a hard brush, but will still provide the benefit of exfoliation.
- The assimilation of nutrients, such as minerals that are contained in seaweed wraps or skin lotions, is improved.
- Lymph and blood circulation are stimulated.
- Nerve-end fibres are rejuvenated.
- Sweat and oil glands are stimulated, restoring moisture and suppleness to the skin.

Right: Polysaccharides in seaweed moisturize the skin.

THALASSOTHERAPY

Derived from the Greek word 'thalassa', which means sea, thalassotherapy is a form of hydrotherapy that incorporates seawater and seaweed into treatments. Earliest references to seaweed treatments go back to early Greek and even Chinese literature. Although France is the main country to have developed modern thalassotherapy at its many resorts, it has also been adopted in recent years by many other countries.

Marine algae in the form of brown, green and red seaweeds are an integral part of the treatments. An interesting characteristic of seaweed is that it absorbs heavy metals readily, so it is important for it to be harvested from unpolluted waters. With

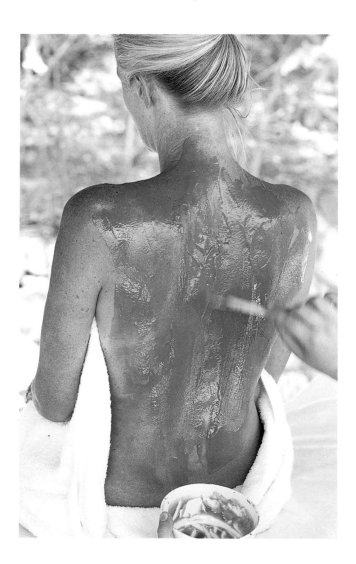

numerous oil spills, as well as pollution of seawater with cadmium, mercury and arsenic, there are unfortunately relatively few places in the world today where seaweed can be harvested safely.

Seaweed products may be used in the form of micronized powders, gels and pastes, or seaweed extracts. The laminaria species, in particular, provide a rich source of vitamins and minerals that are absorbed through the skin during treatments. Iodine is an important component that increases metabolic rate, and enhances detoxification and weight loss.

A typical thalassotherapy treatment starts with exfoliation and a body scrub, followed by underwater massage in a bath that contains seawater or seaweed extract added to ordinary water. The underwater massage has the effect of promoting lymphatic drainage. A seaweed wrap follows, during which time profuse sweating occurs. Before showering off the seaweed you need to drink a glass of water to replace fluid loss.

Contra-indications to the use of seaweed products and seaweed wraps include iodine sensitivity, an overactive thyroid and high blood pressure.

What are its anti-ageing benefits?
1. Metabolic rate increases and weight loss is enhanced.
2. Detoxification and elimination of waste products is promoted.
3. It has all the benefits of hydrotherapy, including being an excellent way to reduce stress.
4. Seaweed contains polysaccharides, which have a moisturizing effect on the skin. The skin feels smooth and silky afterwards.

OTHER BENEFITS FROM THE SEA
In addition to body treatments, seaweed (kelp) capsules are rich in minerals and good for promoting healthy hair, as well as weight loss. Sea vegetables such as Nori, Kombu and Wakame are now freely available in the West. Low in calories and full of nutrients, sea vegetables are a good source of protein, magnesium, folate, vitamin A, vitamin C, iodine and calcium. Seaweed capsules and treatments should not be used by anyone who is iodine sensitive. Kelp capsules, taken together with a zinc supplement, can be used to treat marginal or subclinical thyroid underactivity (*see* thyroid test, page 19).

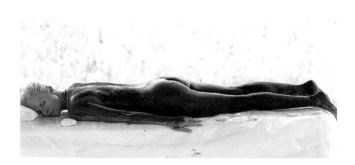

Above and left: Seaweed, combined with mud, is applied to the whole body, which is later wrapped in plastic. This helps to increase the metabolism and promote both fluid loss and detoxification.

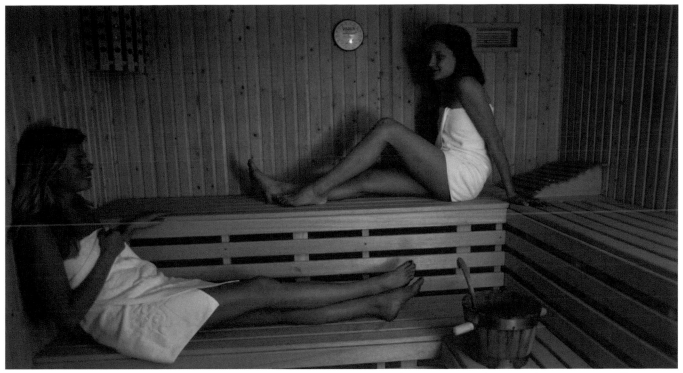

Sauna bathing releases beta-endorphins or 'happiness hormones', reduces stress and generally promotes wellbeing.

THE SAUNA

The medical effects of sauna baths have been studied scientifically for at least two centuries. The UKK Sports Science Institute in Tampere, Finland, has produced numerous papers on sauna bathing, which is such an integral part of every Finn's health maintenance programme. However, sauna bathing is not originally a Finnish invention. It has its origins in Eastern and early Roman bathing cultures. In Turkey, we find the exotic 'hamman', whereas the Romans incorporated a 'caldarium' into their day spas or bathhouses. Splendidly decorated modern versions of hammans and caldariums have become popular in today's health resorts and spas. They incorporate fragrant aromatherapy oils to enhance the body-mind relaxing effect and are guaranteed to cause an outpouring of endorphins, or happiness hormones.

Alcohol causes a fall in blood pressure, so never drink alcohol before having a sauna. In fact, the term 'Finnish roulette' is applied to someone who consumes alcohol just before taking a sauna and then dives into an icy-cold lake.

Another contra-indication is strenuous exercise that revs up the metabolism. It is not advisable to sauna immediately after working out in the gym; rather cool off for 20 to 30 minutes before entering the sauna.

Sauna bathing is safe for people with high blood pressure, as long as it is well controlled. Those with heart problems should not have a cold shower afterwards, but shower with lukewarm water.

The Finns talk about 'loyly', which means that all the conditions regarding correct temperature and humidity inside the sauna are perfect. They also focus on the spiritual experience of sauna bathing, saying that you should behave inside the sauna as if you are in a church. It is a Finnish custom for people to beat themselves with a birch whisk to stimulate sweating and circulation. Some bathers even complete their ritual by hugging a (birch) tree.

The question many people ask is: 'Which is more beneficial – a sauna or a steam bath?' They have similar effects but in general the steam bath temperatures are lower, so the effects are less pronounced.

What are its anti-ageing benefits?

Sauna bathing is beneficial for both body and mind.

1. Heat exposure greatly increases the superficial circulation.
2. Heart rate is increased, metabolism is revved up, and changes occur similar to those that occur with physical exercise.
3. Sweating results in toxins being released through the skin. Sauna bathing is one of the methods used for detoxification of the liver and fat-soluble toxins – for example, if a person has accidentally ingested industrial chemicals. In addition, about 1kg (about 2 lb) of weight loss occurs as a result of sweating.
4. There is a significant increase in beta-endorphins, which accounts for the agreeable sensation of wellbeing after a sauna. As a result, sauna bathing is good for reducing stress levels.
5. Regular sauna bathing helps to enhance the immune system.
6. Muscles are relaxed and rheumatic symptoms are relieved.
7. It facilitates peaceful sleep.
8. Cold water showering or bathing following a sauna helps to stimulate thermogenesis, or fat burning, by the brown adipose tissue. Brown adipose tissue is found in small amounts in the body, but is an important metabolically active area that burns calories.

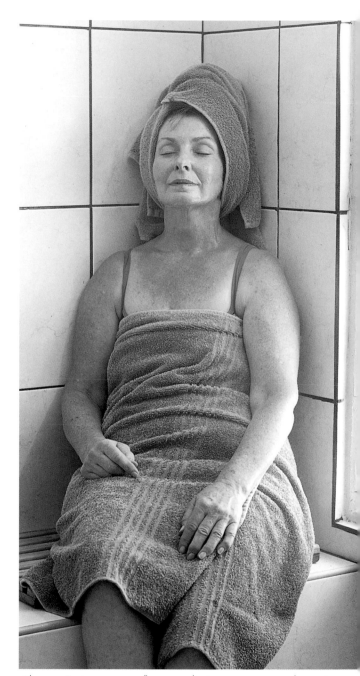

Above: A steam room (hamman) gives a more gentle, moist heat than a sauna but has similar benefits. It increases superficial circulation, stimulates metabolism, releases stress-reducing endorphins and promotes wellbeing.

Left: Correct sauna temperature and humidity are important. Alternating heat with showering or plunging into cold water stimulates fat burning.

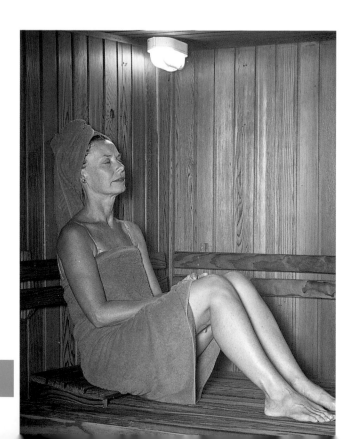

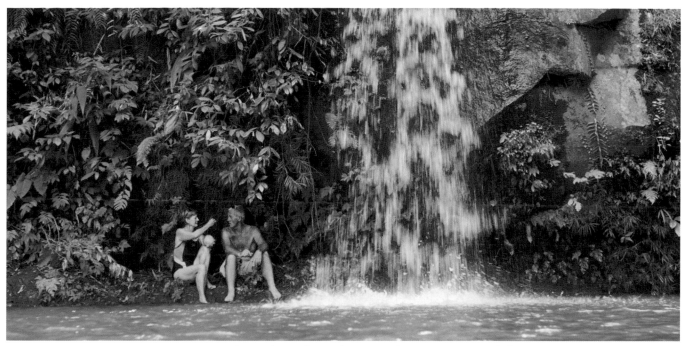

Energizing negative air ions promote vitality – if you do not live near the sea or a waterfall, simply take a daily shower.

NEGATIVE AIR ION THERAPY

How do you feel after taking a bracing walk along the beach next to the pounding surf, or with waves crashing on the rocks? Do you feel revitalized? You should be feeling the energizing effect of negative air ions in the atmosphere. Negative air ions are generated next to moving water. They occur when there is good wave action at the seaside, or when you are standing next to a waterfall, or a fountain, after a thunderstorm, and even while standing under a shower in your bathroom.

By contrast, you will probably have experienced the enervating effect of positive air ions in the atmosphere. They occur just before a thunderstorm or with certain warm winds such as the Mistral in France, the Foehn in Austria, the Santa Ana in Southern California, the Chinook in Canada, the Sharov in Israel, and the Berg wind in southern Africa. These winds generally make you feel tired, irritable and unproductive.

Although it is possible to buy an ionizer for use in your office, your car, or your home, a good way to obtain your daily dose of negative ions is to have a shower, preferably after exercise so that your body is really warm. You can then enjoy the added benefit of the Kneipp method of taking a warm shower, followed by a cold shower to rev up your circulation and immune system.

A mass of scientific research, mainly from Russia, the United States, Germany and the United Kingdom, has shown that negative air ions:
- Protect against stress, as well as lowering irritability and tension
- Improve neurological disorders
- Act as an antidepressant
- Enhance recovery after strenuous exercise
- Improve memory, mood and performance

Negative air ions are increased:
- At the seaside
- In mountain air, and next to waterfalls or fountains
- After a storm
- Under a shower
- By ionizer machines
- When walking barefoot on wet grass

Positive air ions are increased:
- Before storms
- When warm winds blow
- By high levels of soil radioactivity
- By computers, air conditioning, electric blankets and all electrical machines

What are the effects on body and mood?

In his book, *Ionisation, Santé, Vitalité*, Dr. Hervé Robert summarizes some of the beneficial effects of negative ions.
- Exercise performance is improved; there is more energy and less fatigue.
- Brain serotonin levels decrease, with relief of both anxiety and depression.
- Increased alpha activity results in better brain wave synchronization, as well as improved mental functioning.

ANTI-AGEING BODY TREATMENTS

As we grow older there is a decline in many parts of our bodies. This decline may occur slowly and be minimal or, with a destructive lifestyle, it may be fast and rather brutal in its effects.

In the same way that you would tend a garden by pulling out weeds before they become a problem, there is a wide range of preventive, therapeutic and enjoyable body treatments that can be used to manage age-related problems such as joint stiffness, muscular aches and pains, and poor circulation.

Massage

Massage, whether it is Swedish or any other variety, is a body-mind therapy par excellence, guaranteed to send you home floating on a cloud of endorphins – unless, of course, you are one of the few people who do not enjoy being touched.

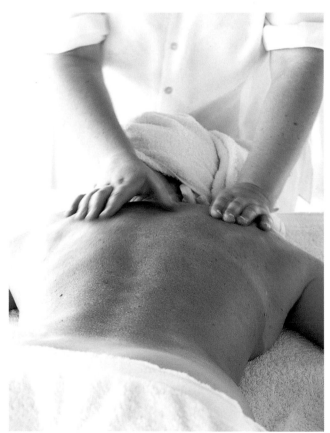

Knuckling uses circular movements and is ideal for massaging feet, hands and shoulders.

The friction method of massage uses the pad of the index finger or thumb. It works well on shoulder muscles.

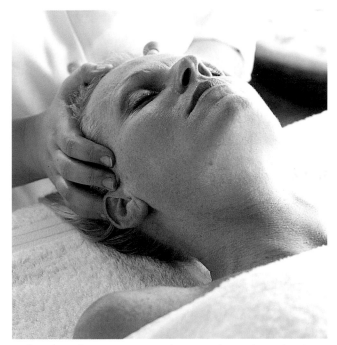

Indian head massage stimulates scalp and cerebral circulation, as well as relaxing tight muscles.

Massage is a most beneficial anti-ageing therapy. It improves circulation, activates and drains lymphatics, and relaxes muscles. Therapeutic massage has been shown to hasten recovery after serious illnesses such as heart attacks, and after surgery and injuries. Massage is also beneficial for stress-related disorders, anxiety, depression and insomnia.

The lymphatic system, consisting of up to a thousand lymph nodes in the body, acts as a filtering system. Lymph carries toxins and waste products away from tissues and organs into the blood stream, from where they are filtered through the liver. The more toxic you are, and the less exercise you perform, the more stagnation occurs in the lymphatic system. Apart from your regular detox diet, exercise and drinking plenty of water, massage assists in draining superficial lymphatics into the deeper vessels, which, in turn, drain into the major blood vessels.

Massage can be applied to specific parts of the body. For instance, Indian head massage improves circulation to the scalp and cerebral vessels, whereas the abdominal massage that forms part of the Austrian 'Mayr cure' targets the gastro-intestinal tract and improves bowel transit time.

What are the benefits?
- Improves lymphatic drainage
- Improves circulation
- Relaxes muscles
- Assists drainage of toxins
- Beta-endorphin release is beneficial for anxiety, depression, insomnia and stress-related disorders

Mud therapy
Italian spas, such as those in Ischia, Abano and Montecatini, use heated mud as applications for rheumatism and fibromyalgia, arthritis and joint stiffness. Known as 'fango', the mud contains microalgae, giving it a greenish-brown colour. Black mud applications used at the Dead Sea resorts in Israel are of benefit in treating musculoskeletal problems. The mud is heated to approximately 40°C (104°F) and has the ability to retain heat, which enhances its therapeutic effects.

In southern Germany and Austria, Moor therapy is used for a wide variety of health problems ranging from arthritis and rheumatism to skin problems. It is also used as an anti-stress and anti-ageing treatment. Moor is a form of organic material created by

Full-body mud baths are of benefit for skin disorders. They also improve joint pain and stiffness.

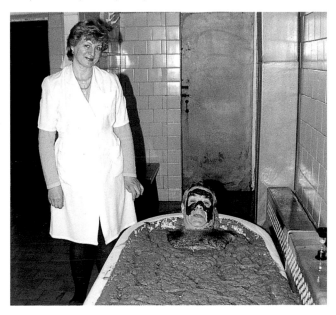

the gradual decomposition of plant matter in an aqueous environment. Over many years, it is transformed into a homogenous dark-brown or black substance that, like other muds, can retain heat over an extended period. When applied to specific problem areas of the body, it increases blood flow, aiding in the healing process. Moor treatments are used for musculoskeletal problems, poor circulation, obesity and skin disorders such as eczema.

If you wish to experience mud treatments you can travel to Europe or Israel, you can have Moor baths at local spas that import the products, or you can purchase home kits that will provide a limited amount for application to specific parts of the body.

What are the benefits?

- With local application, blood flow is increased to problem areas to enhance healing.
- Application of heat creates muscle relaxation, with improvement in joint pain and stiffness.
- Plant ingredients in Moor mud are also beneficial for skin disorders.

Acupressure and shiatsu

With the application of firm fingertip pressure to acupuncture points, the meridians or 'energy channels' in the body are unblocked, facilitating the flow of 'Qi' or vital energy. For those who are not familiar with the concepts of Chinese medicine, it is important to know that one of the most basic principles is that of the body's energy and the fact that it runs through the body in a number of channels, or meridians. An enormous amount of research has been conducted on acupuncture, most of it in Chinese. Western doctors may be sceptical, but the Chinese have successfully used acupuncture and the concept of meridians for at least three thousand years; they do not need to prove themselves to the West.

To the Western mind the concept of Qi may be difficult, but think about how sometimes you are aware that your energy levels are low, whereas at other times you are literally bursting with energy. This is Qi, or what is known as the body's vital energy.

Shiatsu is the Japanese form of acupressure and works on similar principles.

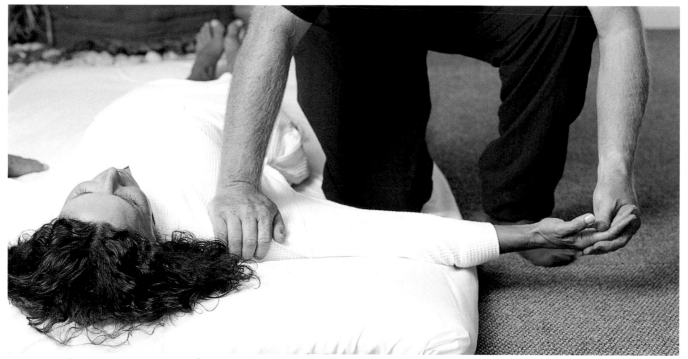

Shiatsu is the Japanese version of acupressure. It applies firm pressure on acupressure points to unblock the energy channels or 'meridians', which facilitates the flow of energy throughout the body.

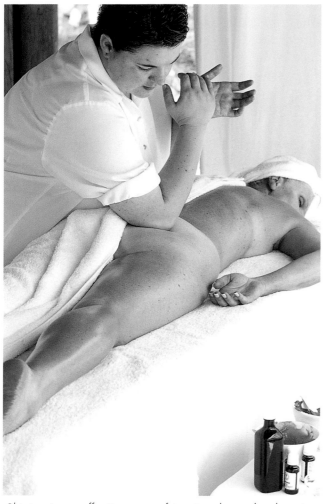

Shiatsu is an effective way of treating lower back pain.

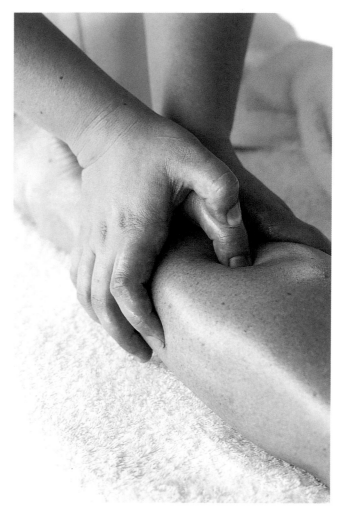

Acupressure on the calf relieves back pain.

What are the benefits?

- The anti-ageing benefits of acupressure/shiatsu include improved blood circulation, as well as overall better co-ordination and functioning of the body's organs.
- According to which meridian is treated, headaches, indigestion, musculoskeletal problems, constipation and general debility can be relieved.
- Treatments are used as part of preventive health care and to keep the body in harmony with the environment, but there are also certain first-aid applications. For example, leg cramps can be relieved by deep pressure between the base of the big toe and second toe for 10 to 15 seconds.

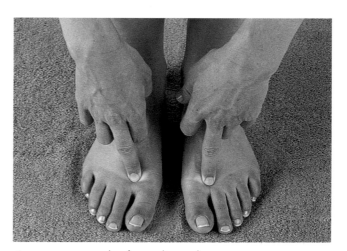

Acupressure on the feet relieves leg cramps.

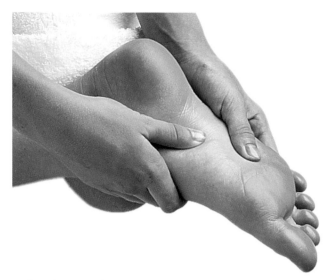

Reflexology involves pressure on specific areas of the foot to treat headaches, digestive problems, and so on.

- Reflexology is a combination of massage and acupressure. It is believed that stimulation of a specific zone on the foot or hand affects other parts of the body. Therapists can treat migraines, digestive problems and various aches and pains. Reflexology is also useful in creating relaxation in older people with neurodegenerative disorders, such as senile dementia and Parkinson's disease.

REFLEXOLOGY

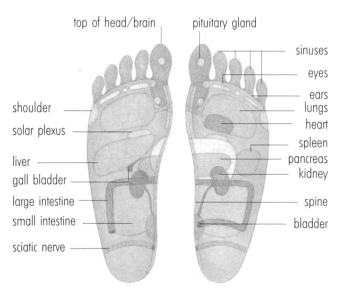

top of head/brain   pituitary gland

sinuses

eyes

ears
lungs
heart

spleen
pancreas
kidney

shoulder

solar plexus

liver

gall bladder

large intestine

small intestine

sciatic nerve

spine

bladder

Manipulation

There are many manipulative therapies, including chiropractic, osteopathy, cranial-sacral osteopathy, polarity therapy, and the Bowen technique to mention just a few.

Chiropractic is a skill in which joints are mobilized in order to obtain relief from back pain, neck pain and other musculoskeletal disorders that commonly occur as we grow older. Instead of taking analgesics or anti-inflammatory drugs, a few minutes of manipulation by a skilled chiropractor may be all that is needed to abolish pain and discomfort.

Below: Chiropractic manipulation creates instant relief from back and neck pain by means of spinal realignment and joint mobilization.

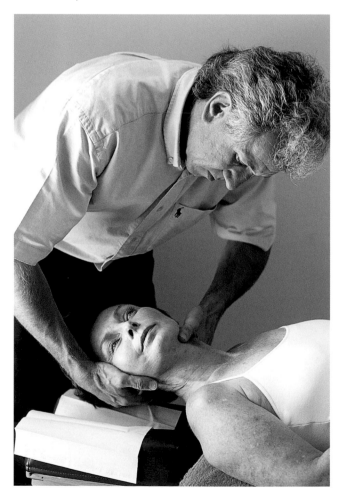

Osteopathy is a system of manipulation of the body and spine to heal the body, even when the signs and symptoms are apparently unrelated. Conceived in the United States by Dr Andrew Still more than a century ago, osteopathy works on several levels, aimed at normalizing function of body parts. Apart from back pain, other problems such as asthma and headaches can be alleviated. Osteopaths often combine their discipline with the practice of naturopathy, involving nutrition and the philosophy that as 'nature heals', the body has the inherent ability to heal itself.

Cranio-sacral osteopathy is a gentle treatment using touch to evaluate and affect the cranium or skull, the spinal column and the cerebrospinal fluid that surrounds the brain and protects the spinal cord. It is believed that changes in the cerebrospinal fluid will affect every cell in the body via the connective tissue. The treatment was developed by American osteopath, Dr John Upledger, and is commonly used to treat chronic pain, postoperative problems and sports injuries.

Polarity therapy was developed by chiropractor and osteopath, Randolph Stone. It combines both oriental and Western therapies. Stone's theory is based on the whole body as an energy field, with the spine as the centre. The head and right side of the body represent the positive electrical pole, while the feet and left side of the body represent the negative electrical pole. His theory is similar to both the yin-yang concept of traditional Chinese medicine and the chakra system of Ayurvedic medicine. The aim of this therapy by touch is to create a balance between positive and negative fields.

The Bowen technique, which was developed by Thomas Bowen in Australia, is now being taught and practised internationally. Using small manipulations of specific parts of the body, this technique aims to restore balance and release tension and blocked energy. Symptoms that respond well to Bowen therapy include back pain, sciatica, neck and shoulder pain, and migraines. Seemingly simple movements are surprisingly effective.

ACTION PLAN

➤ Practice daily skin brushing using a soft brush.

➤ Have a warm shower, followed by a cold shower, daily – preferably after exercise when your body is thoroughly warmed.

➤ Make time for regular massage.

➤ For those backaches and muscular aches and pains, try acupressure or manipulation before you take analgesics or anti-inflammatory drugs.

➤ If you have never experienced hydrotherapy or thalassotherapy – give yourself a treat. They have a powerful anti-ageing effect.

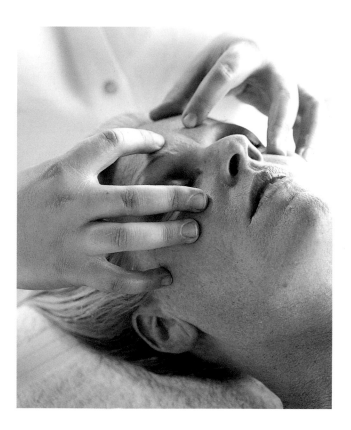

Left: Cranio-sacral osteopathy is a gentle technique to treat chronic pain and postoperative disability.

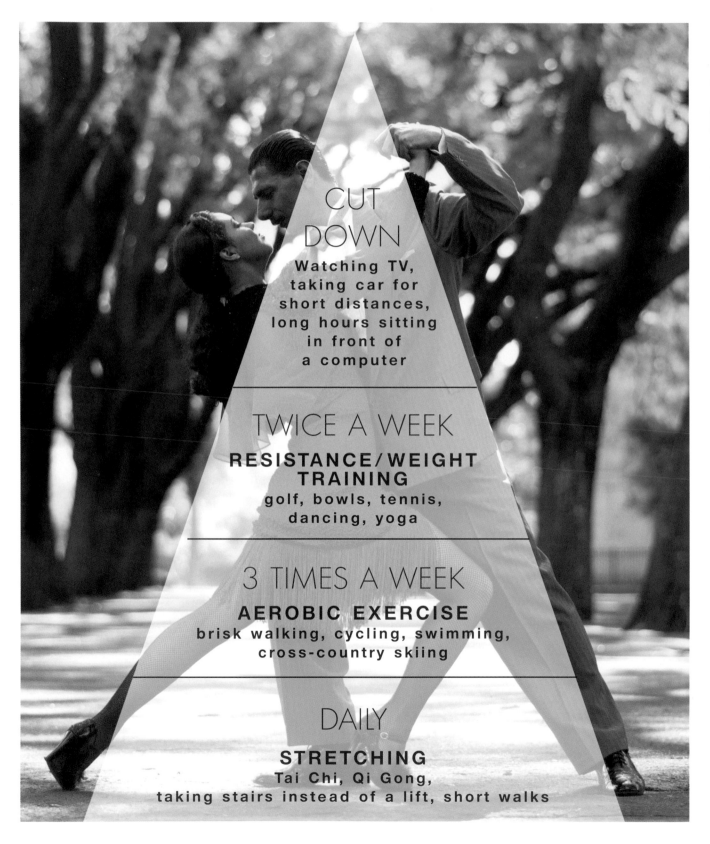

CUT
DOWN
Watching TV,
taking car for
short distances,
long hours sitting
in front of
a computer

TWICE A WEEK
**RESISTANCE/WEIGHT
TRAINING**
**golf, bowls, tennis,
dancing, yoga**

3 TIMES A WEEK
AEROBIC EXERCISE
**brisk walking, cycling, swimming,
cross-country skiing**

DAILY
STRETCHING
**Tai Chi, Qi Gong,
taking stairs instead of a lift, short walks**

THE EXERCISE PYRAMID

KEEP IN SHAPE

The days of 'no pain, no gain' are over. When we talk about exercise for healthy ageing this does not mean that we should indulge in strenuous activities. Apart from anything else, we know that strenuous exercise generates free radicals that can hasten the ageing process if there are insufficient antioxidants to counteract them. If you are to initiate or continue physical exercise, and you intend carrying on with that exercise for the next few decades, it is vital that you choose activities that you enjoy – activities that are not boring, have variety and fit in with your daily routine.

You are at your peak at age 35. After that there is a slow decline, but the good news is that with appropriate exercise, you can do something to halt and even reverse the process.

EVALUATING YOUR FITNESS

For those of you who have medical problems, such as high blood pressure or diabetes, see your doctor before embarking on a fitness programme. If you have never exercised before and you are over 40, you should also have a medical checkup before you start to exercise in a gym.

If you were previously fit, but now have not exercised for several months or even years, it is alarming to know that without exercise you will lose 50 per cent of your fitness. However, if you start training at least three times a week, you will regain that fitness.

At this point in your life, whether you are 40 or 60, you need an honest evaluation of your fitness level. How do you do this?

The easiest way is to have a fitness test at your local gym. You will be tested for body composition and body fat, cardiovascular fitness, muscular strength and flexibility. If this facility is not available, you can test yourself.

- Can you walk up four flights of steps without feeling breathless?
- Can you lift a 20kg (44 lb) suitcase as easily as you did when you were 35?
- Can you sit on the floor with your legs straight and touch your toes?

If you are not used to regular exercise you should always test yourself before you start your programme, then do regular checks every three months to assess progress. It is really motivating to monitor improvement. Make a graph with your weight plotted against weeks and months. Weigh yourself once a week. Do not be upset if you actually gain weight during the first two months of muscle strengthening – you will be losing fat and gaining muscle. Muscle weighs more than fat, which will account for your weight remaining static or temporarily increasing. You will, however, change shape, losing that 'middle-aged spread' in the abdominal area.

The average percentage fat for a middle-aged woman is 30 per cent; for a middle-aged man it is 22 per cent to 25 per cent. You will not be able to measure body fat at home unless you have skin calipers or one of those special scales, but you can do the next best thing, which is to measure your body mass index (BMI), your waist measurement and your waist to hip ratio.

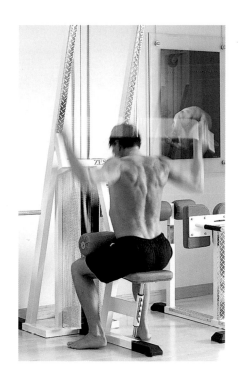

Exercising back muscles

	BMI	WAIST IN CM	WAIST TO HIP RATIO
Normal female	18–25	< 80cm	
Overweight female	> 25	> 80cm	
Obese female	> 30	> 88cm	> 0.85
Normal male	18–25	< 94cm	
Overweight male	> 25	> 94cm	
Obese male	> 30	> 102cm	> 1.0

Remember that in Chapter Two, we looked at how to calculate BMI, with the following formula:

BMI = weight in kg ÷ square of height in metres

(Note: BMI uses metric measurements. To convert pounds to kilograms, divide by 2.2; to convert inches to metres, multiply by 0.0254.)

Method to measure the waist to hip ratio:
• The waist circumference is the shortest circumference measured halfway between the lower rib margin and the iliac crest (top of your hip bone).
• The hip circumference is taken at the top of your thigh bone.
• The waist to hip ratio is calculated as the ratio between the waist and hip circumference.
• An increased waist-hip ratio is related to increased risk of Syndrome X (*see* page 21), heart disease, diabetes and high blood pressure.

After your initial evaluation, take a good look at yourself naked in front of a full-length mirror. Are you happy with what you see?

If you are satisfied, you obviously practise regular exercise, but maybe even you need some fine-tuning. The primary concern here should be prevention of age-related bodily decline. If you are overweight, however, try to focus on the concept of metabolic fitness rather than your weight in kilograms or pounds. After you have achieved fitness, the weight loss should automatically follow.

ESSENTIAL ANTI-AGEING PHYSICAL ACTIVITIES
Aerobic exercise
This means exercise that uses large muscles (leg muscles for walking, and arm muscles for rowing), lasts for at least 15 minutes without stopping, and allows you to breathe deeply but still talk normally. Since aerobic fitness protects the heart, it is also called cardiovascular fitness.

Muscle strengthening
In order to combat age-related loss of muscle, there are various muscle groups in the body that need to be strengthened. The term 'sarcopenia' is used to describe loss of muscle, as well as decreased quality of muscle tissue in older adults.

Flexibility
As you age, ligaments and tendons shorten. This is known as 'adaptive shortening'. If this happens, the joints become stiff and your range of movement becomes limited. Middle-aged people often resort to analgesics for joint pains when they could prevent this simply by stretching. Daily stretching is essential and there is a variety of stretching exercises appropriate for everyday activities, for sports, for the office, or for travelling by plane.

Balance and agility
As you age, you slowly begin to lose your sense of balance and co-ordination. This becomes important in elderly people, who might sustain a fracture if they fall, especially if they are osteoporotic. The good news is that there are specific exercises to improve balance. One of the most enjoyable is ballroom dancing. If you do not know how to samba, perhaps now is the time to learn.

Back exercise
Care of the back is absolutely essential as you age. With degenerative changes of the spinal vertebrae and intervertebral spaces, as well as possible osteoporosis, you need to establish strong abdominal muscles, as well as strengthen the long sacrospinal muscles on either side of the spine in order to support the vertebral column.

Breathing

Everybody breathes in order to live, but so often people do not breathe properly. During your exercise programme, during meditation and relaxation, practise deep abdominal breathing to fill your lungs with revitalizing oxygen.

FOUR RULES OF METABOLIC FITNESS

Having checked your fitness level, the next step is to choose your exercises. For metabolic fitness and body shaping, the following are essential.

1. Aerobic exercise – three to four times a week, lasting for at least 30 minutes
2. Muscle strengthening – three times a week for 20 minutes
3. Stretching – daily
4. Back care – daily or five times a week

Exercise physiologists will tell you to do your aerobic exercise every second day, alternating with muscle strengthening. However, older people may choose a brisk walk every day and incorporate some muscle strengthening into their routine. This routine can be followed whether you are in town or in the country, and no specialized gym equipment is needed. Here is an example of such a programme:

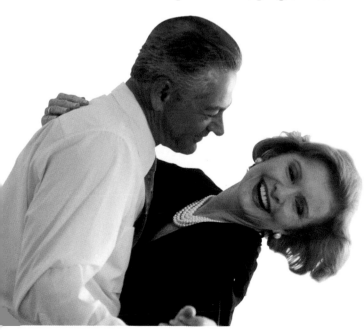

Dancing is a wonderful way to prevent osteoporosis.

Warm-up stretches:	5 minutes
Brisk walk:	30 minutes
Strengthen muscles with elastic bands/tubing:	10 minutes
Stretching and back exercises:	10 minutes
TOTAL:	55 minutes

Stretching should always be performed before and after exercise – a few basic stretches before, and a full body stretch afterwards. Five minutes of back-strengthening exercise can also be incorporated into your stretching routine.

To avoid boredom choose a variety of activities, but always remember to incorporate the four rules of metabolic fitness.

Top five aerobic activities
- Walking
- Cycling
- Swimming
- Racquet sports
- Cross-country skiing

You will notice jogging has not been included as a recommendation for aerobic exercise. Although you may have been jogging in your earlier years, the problem is that stressful weight bearing causes wear and tear of the cartilage in your ankle, knee and hip joints. Increasing age exacerbates degenerative changes. Vigorous walking is the best possible exercise for anyone over the age of 40.

Top five muscle-strengthening activities
- Resistance training in the gym
- Aquacize (*see* page 91)
- Pilates (*see* page 91)
- Elastic bands or tubing (*see* page 89)
- Golf (upper body)

Golf has become a popular pastime and is interesting in that it combines several of the ingredients of good exercise. It is not aerobic, although you may walk fair distances, but it is weight bearing, and requires upper-body strength, flexibility and co-ordination. Your golf performance will be improved by implementing the four basic rules of metabolic fitness.

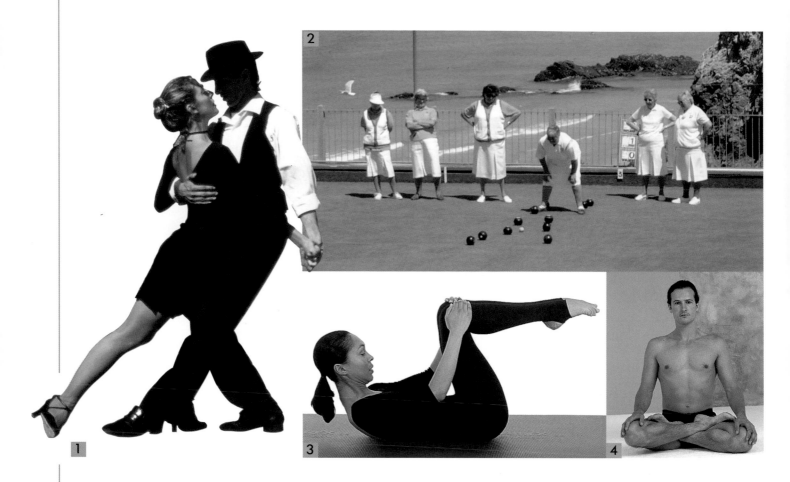

1. Dancing. 2. Bowls. 3. Pilates. 4. Yoga.

Top five activities for balance and co-ordination
- Dancing
- Tai Chi (*see* page 86)
- Alpine skiing
- Bowls/boules/petanque
- Yoga

Weight-bearing exercise to prevent osteoporosis
- Walking (includes golf)
- Dancing
- Rebounding on a mini-trampoline
- Racquet sports
- Stair climbing

Exercises to promote flexibility
- Yoga
- Pilates
- Tai Chi

Exercises to improve posture
- Alexander technique (*see* page 90)
- Pilates

Exercises to improve energy and activate Qi
- Chinese balls (*see* page 87)
- The Five Rites of Rejuvenation (*see* page 88)
- Qi Gong (*see* page 87)
- Swimming in cold water
- Breathing exercises

THE AGEING FRAME	WHAT HAPPENS	WHICH EXERCISE HELPS
Loss of lean body mass	Normal ageing + inactivity results in loss of muscle: 30% loss by age 65 5% loss per decade after 35	Resistance training in gym, elastic tubing, aquacize, Pilates
Loss of aerobic capacity	Couch potatoes lose 35% of cardiovascular fitness by age 65 Decreased speed	Walking, cycling, swimming, cross-country skiing, stair climbing, rowing, racquet sports
Loss of bone mineral density	Osteoporosis Risk of fractures Height loss: 2–4cm ($\frac{3}{4}$–$1\frac{1}{2}$ in) Women lose 35–40% of bone calcium after menopause	Weight-bearing exercises, walking, dancing, rebounding, stair climbing, racquet sports, golf
Flexibility diminishes	Adaptive shortening Ligaments and tendons stiffen, become rigid Pain and stiffness Limited range of movement	Daily stretching exercises, yoga, Pilates, Tai Chi
Loss of agility and balance	Neuromuscular performance diminishes Tendency to fall Slow reaction time 10% decline in nerve conduction time	Dancing, Tai Chi
'Shrinking'/loss of height	Poor posture, stooping 2–4cm ($\frac{3}{4}$–$1\frac{1}{2}$ in) shorter	Alexander technique, Pilates
Backache	Muscles alongside vertebrae become weak Abdominal muscles weak Spine not well supported + degenerative changes in vertebrae	Back exercises to strengthen abdominal muscles, stretching
Body shape changes	Loss of muscle Increase in fat Fat deposited in abdominal area Waist thickens	Aerobic exercise + muscle building exercise + restricted calorie intake
MALE: loss of sexual potency	Testosterone levels drop Andropause	Five Rites of Rejuvenation, aerobic exercise + muscle strengthening + swimming in unheated pool or cold water
FEMALE: genito-urinary ageing	Stress incontinence Lower libido Menopause	Kegel exercises (see page 98), pelvic tilt
Lack of energy Memory loss Fatigue	Premature ageing	Qi Gong, Five Rites of Rejuvenation, breathing exercises, Chinese balls

KEGEL EXERCISES

These strengthening exercises, aimed at tightening the slack vaginal muscles after childbirth, may be practised throughout a woman's adult life. Developed by Dr. Kegel to strengthen the pelvic floor and prevent urinary stress incontinence, they also benefit sexual and orgasmic functioning.

Method: Contract the band of muscles that encircle the vagina. Hold for a count of four.

Repeat five times. Gradually work up to holding the contraction for a count of 10.

An alternative method is to use vaginal cones, which you can get from your gynaecologist. They are inserted into the vagina and held there to work on strengthening the pelvic floor muscles.

THE PELVIC TILT

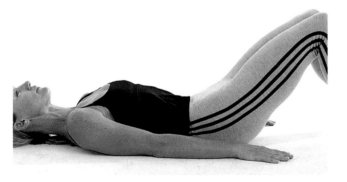

Pelvic tilt is used to strengthen pelvic muscles and should be used together with Kegel exercises. Lie flat with knees bent (above). Slowly lift buttocks just off the floor (below).

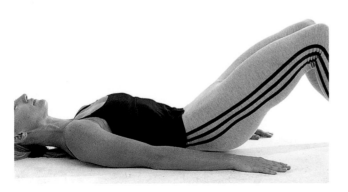

EXERCISE TO TURN BACK THE CLOCK

Sedentary people age quickly and develop changes in body composition and loss of function as shown in the table on page 85. By contrast, studies have shown that active men of 55 years maintain the same blood pressure, weight and aerobic capacity as they had aged 40. A 30-minute brisk walk performed by an older person three or four times a week can turn back the biological clock by some 10 years.

Research also shows that people of 60 and 70 who exercise regularly can achieve fitness levels associated with men and women 20 to 30 years younger. Improvements have been noted in muscular strength, body composition, joint flexibility, lung function, heart disease risk profile, osteoporosis prevention and enhanced resistance to depression. Exercise results in an outpouring of your happiness hormones, the beta-endorphins. This is a cost-effective, non-pharmacological and life-enhancing method of dealing with depression, which is such a common problem in older men and women.

You are never too old to start an exercise programme. A recent research project involved a group of men and women living in a retirement village. They were all over the age of 85. A three-month programme of muscle strengthening exercises, practised three days a week, resulted in an increase of muscular strength by 75 per cent.

Although disuse causes rapid loss of muscle, this study shows that exercise can rebuild it. The most important appointment that you have each day is your exercise session.

SECRETS FROM THE ORIENT
Tai Chi

This ancient Chinese martial art consists of slow, continuous, smooth and graceful movements executed with suppleness and in a relaxed manner. It is a combination of movement, balance, mental relaxation and correct breathing.

Tai Chi is an ideal exercise for older people. You will almost never see an overweight middle-aged or elderly Chinese person: at the age of 80, they are still active members of the household, and can be seen practising their early morning Tai Chi exercises in a park near to their homes.

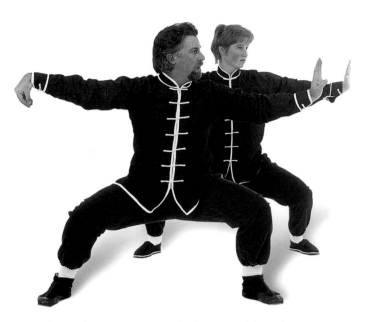

Tai chi combines movement, balance and breathing.

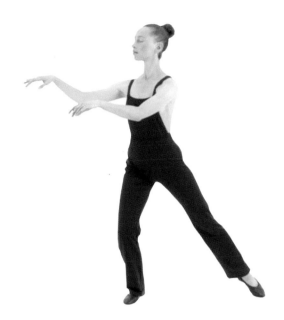

Qi Gong promotes mental relaxation and clarity.

Tai Chi exercises the cardiovascular system. A 30-minute Tai Chi workout would be equivalent to a three-hour game of golf. Joints are loosened and co-ordination improved. At first, you will need lessons with a teacher, after which you can spend 10 minutes each day in your own home or garden, practising this enjoyable form of activating your body's energy levels.

Qi Gong

Pronounced Chi Kung, this Chinese exercise is a combination of breathing, meditation and very slow and controlled movements.

How does Qi Gong differ from Tai Chi? They both act by increasing your Qi or inner energy levels, but Qi Gong incorporates much less movement and more mental concentration. It can be described as 'moving meditation'. The movements are very slow and gentle, and you need to be calm and centred while performing them. Scientific studies recording electro-encephalogram (EEG) brain waves of subjects practising Qi Gong show that there is a shift towards theta brain waves, which are associated with deep meditation, rather than the beta waves usually associated with day-to-day living.

Your Qi Gong teacher will probably have experience in Tai Chi as well. Qi Gong movements are simple and you will soon be able to practise them at home. Try to do them for 15 minutes every day. You will not experience immediate results, but after one or two months you will experience an increase in energy, mental clarity and emotional wellbeing.

Chinese balls

These balls are used to improve arm circulation and hand co-ordination. They also activate acupressure points on the palms of the hands, thus activating your inner energy. They are often used by middle-aged and elderly Chinese people as a part of their overall preventive health regime.

Hold two matching balls, about 4cm (1½ in) in diameter, in one hand. Rotate the balls slowly in one direction, then change to the opposite direction. If you do not have Chinese balls, you can use chestnuts or even golf balls.

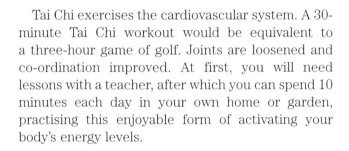

The Five Rites of Rejuvenation

Also known as 'The Five Tibetans' (*see* page 124), these yoga exercises have a romantic history. In the 1930s, a British army colonel stationed in India heard about lamas from a particular monastery in Tibet who had discovered the 'secret of the fountain of youth'. These rites were reputed to strengthen the body, enhance energy, regenerate body and mind, and stem the ageing process. The colonel searched and found the monastery. After spending some time there, he himself experienced a feeling of marked rejuvenation and enhanced vitality.

What was the monks' secret?

The lamas were mainly vegetarian, did not overeat, and practised food combining (which, in fact, is food separating). They also meditated and generally led a stress-free existence.

The five exercises they practised daily involved twisting, turning and stretching, activating energy points and energy channels in the body. Thus, it was a combination of factors that kept them remarkably youthful. The colonel made a relevant comment: 'If you are able to visualize yourself as young, others will see you that way too.' Renowned author, Deepak Chopra, has basically the same advice when he writes about reversing your biological age by changing perceptions of your body.

How do the Five Rites promote longevity?

Their purpose is to influence the energy channels in your body so that they can function at peak activity. Each exercise stimulates various nerve endings that lie along the vertebral column. The Chinese energy system runs through 'meridians', whereas the Indian and Tibetan energy systems connect through 'chakras', which are the seven energy centres in the body. The systems are similar in that they recognize the fundamental concept of energy.

How do you practise the Five Rites?

You should receive instruction from an experienced yoga teacher before attempting the exercises alone. Start slowly with three repetitions, and build up to the recommended 12 repetitions daily. The exercises should be practised on an empty stomach, wearing loose clothing. Some of them will be difficult for people with arthritis or lower back problems. They should not be practised by the over-sixties who have never done yoga before – unless they are supervised and proceed very slowly at first. This is in contrast to Tai Chi and Qi Gong, which can be enjoyed safely whether you are 40 or 80.

Tai Chi, Qi Gong and the Five Rites are all psycho-physical exercises that have a number of benefits in common.
- They create balance and harmony in thought and action.
- They improve circulation.
- They lower cortisol and stress levels.
- They improve breathing.
- They improve balance and co-ordination.
- They encourage flexibility and help to combat joint stiffness.

You may feel reluctant to practise Eastern exercises, but they have been included in this book because they are ideal for older people and can be practised in the privacy of your home without the need for special equipment. The exercises are not aerobic, so they should not be your only form of exercise but rather part of your overall fitness programme. An ideal companion to these exercises would be to walk for 30 minutes every day.

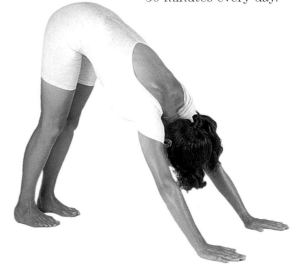

The Five Rites are yoga exercises that activate energy points and energy channels in the body.

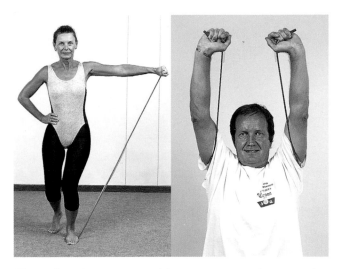

Elastic bands are a portable way to strengthen muscles.

ELASTIC BANDS

Also known as 'therabands' or 'dynabands', these consist of lengths of rubber tubing or sheets of rubber of different strengths. You can purchase a set at your local sports shop, which will include an instruction book of exercises. You can even ask your local pharmacy to supply you with one metre of surgical tubing for exactly the same effect. Exercising with elastic bands or tubing has the dual benefit of both strengthening and stretching muscles. If you are travelling away from home you can take your tubing with you – ideal for those business trips or holidays.

STRETCHING

Nothing is more important for the maintenance of a youthful body than a daily session of stretching. The older you get, the more important it becomes. You need to maintain and improve your current level of flexibility otherwise you will become stiffer

Right: Without daily stretching, adaptive tendon shortening leads to limited movement and joint stiffness.

and stiffer as time passes and adaptive shortening of tendons and ligaments begins. Stretching helps to prevent injuries and muscle strains. It also makes all kinds of exercises easier.

There is a right way and a wrong way to stretch. It can be harmful if you bounce or stretch until you feel pain. When you begin a stretch, take it easy, and go to a point where you feel just a mild degree of resistance. Hold for about 15 seconds. Then start with a second stretch, slowly moving a little further. Hold for 15 seconds. Do not hold your breath while stretching; breathe in and out easily.

When should you stretch?

In general, it is a good idea to do some gentle stretches relevant to the exercise you are about to start, but your main series of stretches can be performed after exercise, when your body and muscles are warm. You can benefit from stretching while sitting at your office desk, in front of the TV, or during a long journey by plane.

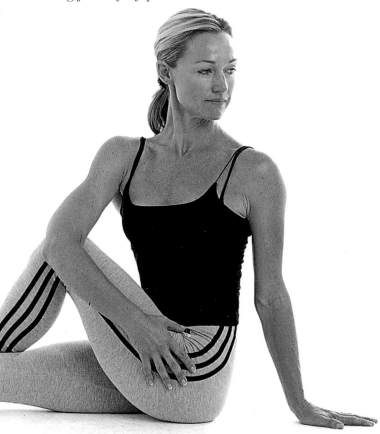

POSTURE

The position of your head is important for achieving correct alignment. Too many older people stand and walk with the head in a forward position. Try to get into the habit of pulling back from what you are doing, and standing tall. Visualize a half-kilogram bag of sugar on your head, and push it towards the ceiling keeping your chin tucked in. Here is a good exercise for practising standing tall.

- Stand next to a wall with your feet a few inches away from it.
- Bend your knees slightly.
- Press your lower back against the wall (*see* left).
- With your chin level, pull your head back and hold for a count of five. Relax, then repeat the head pull- in three times.

The Alexander technique is a posture training method developed by Australian practitioner Mathias Alexander in 1970. An Alexander technique teacher will help you to rediscover your natural posture and movement patterns by correcting superimposed wrong postures that may induce mental and physical tension. The Alexander method is not a quick fix; it takes time and several sessions of training to achieve results. It is helpful for backache, specific postural problems, migraines, anxiety and tension.

BACK EXERCISES

If you have a back problem, consult a physiotherapist before doing exercises. A good back programme helps to maintain your back in two ways. Firstly, it strengthens the abdominal muscles that support your back. Secondly, it keeps your back flexible. A correctly aligned back helps to ensure good posture.

1. Lie on your back with your knees bent. Tighten your abdominal muscles while tilting the pelvis slightly. Hold this tension for 10 seconds while breathing normally. Repeat three times.
2. Lie on your back with the knees bent. Lift your right knee towards your chest. Keep your lower back flat on the floor and draw the navel towards your spine. Hold the stretch for 10 seconds. Repeat three times with each leg.
3. To stretch the lower back, lie on your back and keep the left leg straight. Bend your right leg and bring it across your body to the left. Hold for 30 seconds. Repeat twice to each side.
4. Lie on your back with arms extended overhead. Stretch arms and legs simultaneously. Pull in your abdominal muscles as you stretch. Hold for five seconds, then relax.

Left: Stand against a wall to correct your posture.
Below: Back exercises strengthen abdominal muscles and the sacrospinal muscles that support your spine. They also promote flexibility and prevent backache.

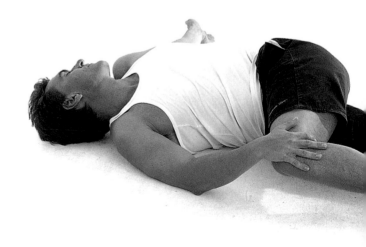

PILATES

Pilates is a series of exercises developed in the early 20th century by the German, Joseph Pilates, to help his own body become stronger. Its purpose is to strengthen, stretch and elongate the muscles. It has been practised by professional dancers and athletes for many years. Pilates combines elements of yoga, breath work and weight training. It can be adapted to men and women of all ages. Apart from floor exercises, teachers may use equipment with exotic names to facilitate exercises, such as 'the reformer', the 'trapeze table', the 'spine corrector', and the 'ladder barrel'. Pilates has recently become fashionable and is indeed a most effective form of exercise. However, since you will have to do it with a teacher in a studio, it will only be available to those living in large towns.

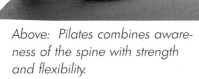

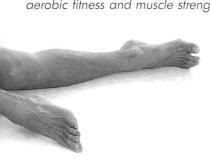

Above: Pilates combines awareness of the spine with strength and flexibility.

Right: Aquacize improves flexibility, aerobic fitness and muscle strength.

AQUACIZE

Exercise in water goes under many names – aquarobics, hydrofit, aquarhythmics are but a few. The pool water is heated to about 30°C (86°F) to create the ideal environment to promote muscle relaxation and flexibility. Aquacize is one of the best types of exercise for older people.

You can take part in aquacize classes with a teacher, which really can be a great deal of fun. Alternatively, you can continue with pool exercises on your own at home if the water in your pool is warm enough.

What are its benefits?

- Aquacize combines aerobic exercise with muscle strengthening.
- It promotes flexibility.
- It is excellent for people who have arthritis or are recovering from knee or hip surgery.
- It is suitable for obese individuals who might have difficulty with other aerobic activities.
- Chances of injury are minimal.

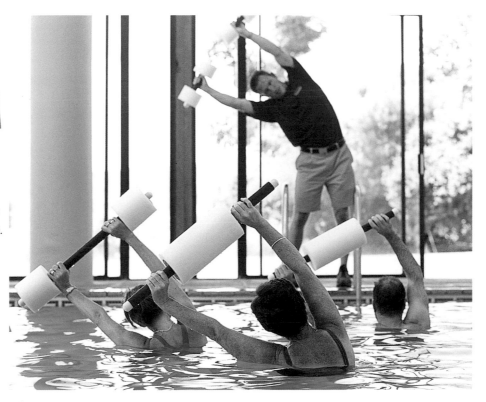

BRITTLE BONES, AGEING AND EXERCISE

The problem of osteoporosis has already been discussed (*see* page 53). A metabolic bone disease characterized by decreased bone density and diminished bone strength, it has become a major health problem in the ageing population. Although it is mainly postmenopausal women who become osteoporotic, men are also at risk if they smoke, consume excessive amounts of alcohol, undergo treatment for prostate cancer, or have low testosterone levels.

What are the risk factors for osteoporosis?

- Lack of exercise, inactivity
- Prolonged bed rest
- A family history
- Menopause and andropause
- Medications: steroids, thyroid replacement, barbiturates, chemotherapy, anti-seizure drugs
- Anorexia, eating disorders
- Cigarette smoking
- Excessive alcohol intake
- Excess consumption of dietary animal protein
- Carbonated drinks

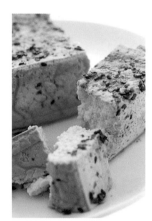

Tofu

How can you prevent osteoporosis?

1. Weight-bearing exercise is the most important way to prevent this disease. Walking, dancing, racquet sports, rebounding on a mini-trampoline and golf all help to keep bones strong and healthy.
2. Diet should contain adequate amounts of calcium and magnesium, but should not include excessive amounts of protein, which results in loss of calcium. Eat soy products such as tofu, but avoid carbonated drinks, because these contain phosphates that combine with calcium and result in loss of calcium from bone.
3. Supplements containing 500–800mg calcium, 300–400mg magnesium, plus boron should be considered from middle age onwards. Soy isoflavone supplements will also help to improve bone mineral density.
4. Oestrogen supplementation for postmenopausal women has been controversial. Although studies have indicated that it does not prevent heart disease, it has been shown that there is 50 per cent reduction in the incidence of hip fractures and 90 per cent decrease in vertebral

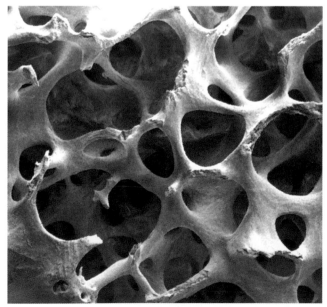

Normal bone is strong and well-mineralized.

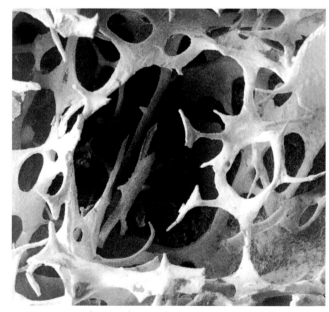

Osteoporotic bone shows decreased mineral density.

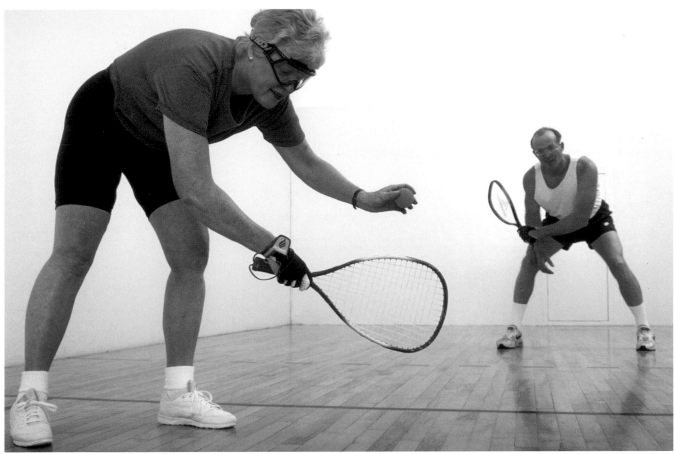

Racquet sports are good for developing aerobic fitness.

fractures in women who take oestrogen supplementation. The dose required to maintain bone mineral density is lower than previously recognized. The recommended dose for transdermal oestrogen, which is delivered through the skin in the form of a gel or patch, is 25 micrograms, and for oral oestrogen it is 0.3mg. Oestrogen also has the benefit of increasing absorption of calcium from the gut. Thus, every woman should decide for herself whether the risks outweigh the benefits of oestrogen.

If your doctor has told you that you have a low bone-mineral density, or that you actually have osteoporosis, what can be done to help? Apart from the points listed above, you may be prescribed medication, such as Raloxifene, biphosphonate compounds or calcitonin nasal spray. Recombinant human parathyroid hormone is being tested, but is not yet approved for general use.

ACTION PLAN

➤ Remember that the most important appointment you have every day is your exercise session.

➤ Evaluate your present fitness level and take pride in monitoring your progress every few months. Make a graph and weigh yourself once a week.

➤ Choose a combination of activities from the suggestions listed, or you may have your own preferred sports. Always include aerobic exercise, muscle strengthening, weight-bearing exercise and daily stretching.

➤ Check your posture.

NUTRITION
good fats,
low-GI foods,
water

SUPPLEMENTS
antioxidants
omega-3s,
B vitamins

HORMONES

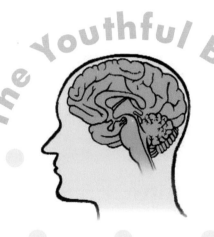

The Youthful Brain

PHYSICAL EXERCISE
brain gym,
aerobic activities

RIGHT AND LEFT
BRAIN BALANCING

MENTAL STIMULATION
bridge,
reading,
mind mapping

MIND-BODY EXERCISES
meditation,
Tai Chi,
Qi Gong

STRESS REDUCTION
sleep,
laughter,
music

THE YOUTHFUL BRAIN

We have now come to the most vital part of your youthful ageing programme – your brain. The wonderful news is that there is so much that you can achieve by following the instructions in this chapter. You can think yourself younger, you can prevent degenerative disorders, and you can improve and enhance your memory.

Your brain is your most precious possession: it houses your personality, your intelligence, your creativity, your rational thinking, your mind and your spirituality. It is absolutely no use having a body that functions well if the brain has deteriorated. With increased life expectancy, the incidence of Alzheimer's disease, age-related memory decline and other brain degenerative disorders has increased, becoming a matter of great concern to men and women from middle age onwards.

In the past, we knew very little about brain function. With new imaging techniques in recent years, however, fascinating discoveries have been made in the field of neuroscience. If we have problems anywhere else in the body – for example, the liver – we can take a biopsy and study the cells under a microscope. But we can hardly do that to our brain, which remains protected in its hard shell, rather like a giant walnut.

Now, however, we have positron emission tomography (PET) scanning as a diagnostic tool that can provide clear images of brain anatomy and function, and even identify future pathology by showing altered metabolism. Magnetic resonance imaging (MRI) scans can identify areas of atrophy and degeneration in Alzheimer's disease. Whereas we were previously able to study the brain only by examining post mortem specimens, this means we can now observe live brain cells in

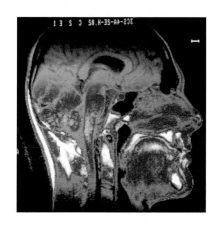

MRI scan of the head showing the brain.

action. Scientists can observe the amount of blood flowing to the brain, and how glucose is used to produce energy.

The human brain weighs an average of 1.4kg, (3 lb) although there are variations of about 500g (1 lb), and a woman's brain weighs at least 50g (1½ oz) less than a man's. If your brain weighs less than the average, does this mean you are less intelligent? Not so: some of the most brilliant historical figures had brains that were only of average weight. For example, Albert Einstein's brain weighed 1.4kg (3 lb), compared to the romantic poet Lord Byron's, which weighed a hefty 2.2kg (5 lb) – yet no one would suggest that Einstein was less intelligent. It is not the size and weight of your brain that is important, but the number of dendrites or tentacles that connect your brain cells.

THE AGEING BRAIN

Nerve cells or neurons communicate with each other by chemical messengers or neurotransmitters (also known as neuropeptides), which spread information throughout the brain. The messages travel along connecting dendrites between the nerve cells. As you age, you steadily lose nerve cells, with about 10–15 per cent loss by the time you are 70, resulting in shrinkage of the brain. The remarkable fact is, however, that by means of mental and physical exercise and correct nutrition, you can actually increase the number of dendrites – and thus connections – between remaining neurons. This means that as you age it is possible for you to prevent memory loss and age-related brain function.

There are an estimated one hundred billion dendritic connections in the human brain. By increasing

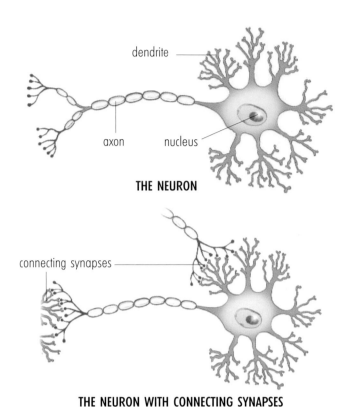

THE NEURON

THE NEURON WITH CONNECTING SYNAPSES

the number of dendrites you can improve your mental capabilities, concentration, motor skills and reaction time. This is wonderful news – and a good example of the old saying: 'Use it or lose it.'

What causes premature brain ageing?

Ageing is accelerated by the wrong foods, by toxins, stress, lack of exercise, lack of stimulation, and by certain medications. The stress hormone, cortisol, interferes with the brain's supply of glucose and with neurotransmitters, resulting in the death of brain cells.

Other brain-ageing factors include:
- Free radicals (the environment, cigarette smoke, ionizing radiation)
- Bad fats, sugar, alcohol, excitotoxins
- Stress, anger, toxic emotions
- Lack of exercise
- Lack of relaxation
- Lack of stimulation
- Drugs or medications
- Lack of oestrogen or testosterone
- Impaired circulation, high blood pressure
- Diabetes

What prevents brain ageing?

If you wish to maintain a youthful brain you need to implement a programme that combines correct nutrition, vitamin and mineral supplementation, physical and mental exercise, and adequate relaxation as well as brain stimulation. It is all part of your youthful ageing lifestyle.

THE BRAIN-BOOSTING PROGRAMME

- Brain food and supplements
- Brain exercise – physical, mental, mind-body
- Brain balancing of right and left sides
- Brain stimulation
- Brain destressing

BRAIN FOOD

In the past it was thought that the brain was not influenced by diet. Today, that assumption has changed. We now know that certain key nutrients – sugars and fats, for instance – have a dramatic impact on brain cells and brain functioning, resulting in mood changes, as well as long-term behavioural changes. We also know that the brain needs the same vitamins and nutrients as the rest of the body, but it needs more of them.

Our ancestors ate a diet consisting of fruit and vegetables, game, fish and whole grains. Today's diet has changed radically. Additives and preservatives, processed and packaged foods, and an abundance of sugar, fats and dairy products comprise a major part of our diet. Aspartame, the artificial sweetener found in diet drinks and desserts, is a powerful excitotoxin that has a cumulative effect, and damages brain cells. Another excitotoxin is the flavour enhancer, monosodium glutamate (MSG), found in sauces, snack foods, Chinese food and packaged soups.

The brain consists of 60 per cent fat, and it is essential that you feed it with the correct type of fat in order for it to function properly. You would hardly put diesel fuel into a car that runs on petrol (gas). So, too, the appropriate fuel is needed for your brain, making the correct fat intake vitally important from early childhood.

We discussed chronic inflammation in Chapter Two (*see* pages 24–25). This applies to the brain as well. If you consume an excess of omega-6 fats, there is persistent inflammation of brain cells, promoting the onset of many neurodegenerative diseases and stroke, as well as general decline of all mental functions. The best advice is for you to cut down on your omega-6 fats, eat more fish and use olive oil for cooking and salad dressings.

Which fats are BAD for your brain?
- Saturated fats found in meat, whole milk, butter and cheese
- Transfatty acids in margarine and fried foods
- Mayonnaise
- An excess of omega-6 vegetable oils, such as sunflower oil

Which fats are GOOD for your brain?
- Omega-3 essential fats found in fish such as salmon, sardines, mackerel, herring, anchovies and trout, as well as fish oil supplements
- Omega-3 fats found in nuts, linseed or flaxseed oil
- Olive oil, a monounsaturated fat

Sugar 'ages' your brain
We have already seen how sugar in the diet combines with proteins by a process known as glycosylation to form sticky compounds called advanced glycosylation end products or AGEs (*see* page 21).

In addition, if your blood sugar levels are too low or too high, your memory is impaired and degenerative diseases can be exacerbated – something that particularly affects older people.

How can you keep blood sugar normal?
- Choose foods with a low glycaemic index (*see* page 52). This includes fruit, vegetables, legumes and whole-grain cereals.
- Avoid high glycaemic index foods. Eat less refined carbohydrates, desserts, sweets and soft drinks.
- Always eat breakfast and have a snack mid-morning and mid-afternoon, but restrict the size of your lunch and dinner. Cutting down the total number of calories promotes longevity, but you need to choose the right foods.
- If you have a problem with fluctuating blood sugar levels, supplementing with chromium, 200 micrograms daily, should help. You may also combine chromium with spirulina to good effect.
- The antioxidant, alpha lipoic acid or ALA (60–100mg daily) protects brain cells and helps with blood sugar control.

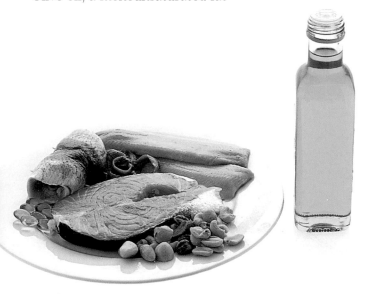

Good fats

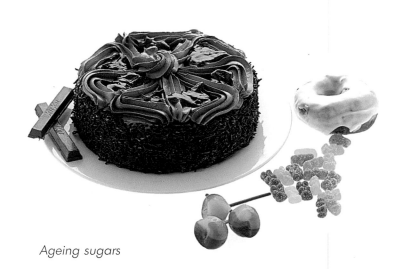

Ageing sugars

OPTIMUM NUTRITION FOR THE BRAIN	
Cut down	**Increase**
Bad fats, omega-6 fats	Omega-3 fats
High glycaemic index foods	Low glycaemic index foods
Size of meals	Number of meals
Alcohol	Water
Excitotoxins (e.g. aspartame, MSG)	Organic fruit and vegetables
Additives, preservatives, packaged and processed foods	Fresh and raw foods

Brain-enhancing supplements

What about supplements? Are there specific supplements to protect the brain, enhance memory, and slow down degenerative processes?

We have identified the fact that the brain requires the same nutrients as the body, but more of them. We also know that the brain thrives on antioxidants and omega-3 fats. Here are some specific supplements suggested for enhancing brain health.

A. Essential
- Vitamin E, 400 units daily
- Vitamin C, 500mg daily
- Flaxseed oil capsules, one daily
- B vitamins: B12, B1, B6, as well as folic acid in combination
- Magnesium, 300mg daily
- Zinc, 20mg daily

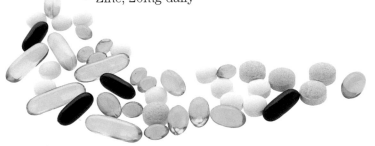

B. Optional
- Alpha lipoic acid, 60–100mg daily, has been shown to protect against neurodegenerative disorders.
- Pycnogenol, derived from pine bark or grape seeds, is a powerful antioxidant.
- Ginkgo biloba, 100mg daily, enhances cerebral circulation.
- Phosphatidyl serine (PS), a naturally occurring form of fat derived from soy, improves memory.
- Acetyl-l-carnitine, which is often used in combination with other 'brain formula' supplements such as PS, is thought to improve your overall mental functioning and memory.

C. Hormones
- DHEA (dehydroepiandrosterone), the adrenal prehormone, decreases with age. As a supplement it is effective in balancing the harmful effects of the stress hormone, cortisol. If your DHEA levels are low and you are suffering from stress, DHEA may be useful. People who have taken DHEA report that they have a definite increase in their feeling of wellbeing.
- Pregnenalone is another prehormone, higher on the hormone cascade. It is derived from cholesterol, but does not have cholesterol's negative effect on the body. It improves memory, and may be included in a multihormone replacement or taken on its own. Both pregnenalone and DHEA should be taken under medical supervision.
- Oestrogen stimulates growth of dendrites and increases the activity of neurotransmitters that send messages across the nerve cells. It also increases circulation and blood flow in the brain. Research has shown that women who take oestrogen as hormone replacement have a 50 per cent lower chance of developing Alzheimer's disease. Research has not yet shown any brain-protecting benefits for women who have decided to take plant or phyto-oestrogens, such as red clover or soy isoflavones. You would thus need to concentrate on brain-enhancing activities as well.
- Testosterone replacement therapy may produce dramatic improvements in wellbeing during the male menopause (andropause), when depression is a major symptom.

PERSONALITY TYPES

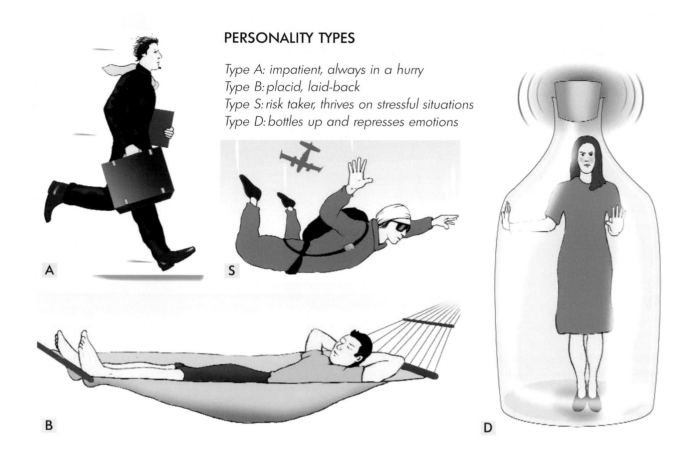

Type A: impatient, always in a hurry
Type B: placid, laid-back
Type S: risk taker, thrives on stressful situations
Type D: bottles up and represses emotions

A

S

B

D

STRESS AND THE BRAIN

Prolonged stress can actually kill brain cells. We have seen that as we age, our stress hormone, cortisol, is the only hormone that increases. This means that older people start off with a raised cortisol level. Once exposed to a stressful emergency or a feeling of anxiety, the normal response is an outpouring of cortisol. However, at the end of the emergency, when levels should be returning to normal, the older person's cortisol levels remain raised.

What about an older person with a Type A personality? This is a term applied to people who respond to neutral situations in a stressful way. They are impatient, hate waiting in queues, become agitated in traffic jams, are subject to 'the hurry syndrome' and often do two activities at the same time. A subgroup of the Type A personality is the person who is hostile or tends to become angry. Hostility is a toxic emotion that damages the heart. With an outpouring of cortisol, it causes damage to the brain as well.

Another personality type is a 'repressive' personality. These people are not hostile or anxious, but successful, hardworking and outwardly happy. However, because they keep a tight lid on their emotions, they have persistently high cortisol levels. In fact, the levels in their bloodstream are as high as those of very anxious people. Repressive personalities are more likely to have cardiac complications, and their permanently elevated cortisol levels are slowly killing off brain cells, putting them at risk of developing memory impairment.

To avoid damaging brain cells as you age, you need to actively adopt measures to lower your cortisol levels. This is part of 'stress management', for which there are techniques everyone needs to learn.

Each individual should choose the method or activities that he or she finds the most convenient and enjoyable. Listening to Mozart, meditating, learning to tango, découpage classes, painting, a weekly massage and sauna bath are all possibilities. Eating healthily and exercising daily are enormously helpful aids to coping with stress.

Make yourself stress resistant

The stress-resistant personality has a number of trademark features.

- A hobby, sport or creative outlet that is practised regularly
- A mind that is relaxed
- The ability to be flexible and adaptable
- The wisdom not to try to control uncontrollable events or situations
- A support group of close relatives or friends

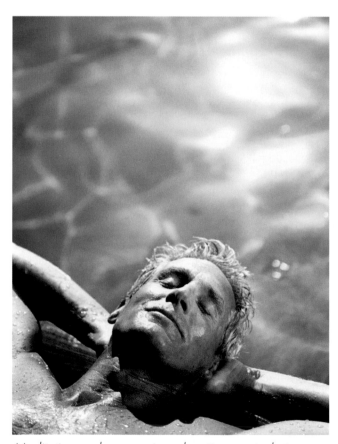

Meditation and progressive relaxation are techniques that lower stress cortisol levels.

Mind-body exercises

'Who can make muddy waters clear?
Let it be still, and it will clear itself.' Lao Tzu

Mind-body exercises include meditation, relaxation, Tai Chi, Qi Gong and yoga, and their common purpose is to quiet the mind.

Meditation can be defined as 'the ability to not think'. Many different techniques can be used to meditate. As a starting point, find time each day to be in a quiet place, lying down or sitting without external disturbances. Then empty your mind – which is often difficult because you will have dozens of intruding thoughts. Repeating a mantra or a particular word may help. Another trick is to focus on your breathing. You may increase your feeling of tranquillity by playing music. Specific tapes for meditation may help to increase the feeling of deep relaxation and peacefulness. Try to spend at least 20 minutes in this relaxed state.

Meditation and deep relaxation have the benefit of lowering stress cortisol levels. The quieting effect on the brain is reflected by electro-encephalograph (EEG) or brainwave studies, which show a shift from the beta waves of normal, day-to-day activity to the more relaxed theta wave activity. Meditation also decreases the pulse rate and blood pressure in people who normally have raised levels.

Another mind-body technique of relieving stress and tension is *progressive relaxation*. Developed by psychologist Edmund Jacobson in the mid-1900s, it has become an integral part of many stress management programmes. It is very simple to practise and you will be surprised to find how much muscular tension you are storing in your body, particularly the neck, shoulders and jaw. This is a good relaxation method for Type A behaviour.

1. Lie down in a quiet, peaceful place.
2. Starting with your toes, gradually move up your body, tensing and then relaxing your muscles.
3. Breathe deeply and slowly. When you have finished, you will be calm and feel as if all your tension has melted away.

Tai Chi and Qi Gong exercises (*see* pages 86–87) can be of considerable benefit to older people and are to be recommended.

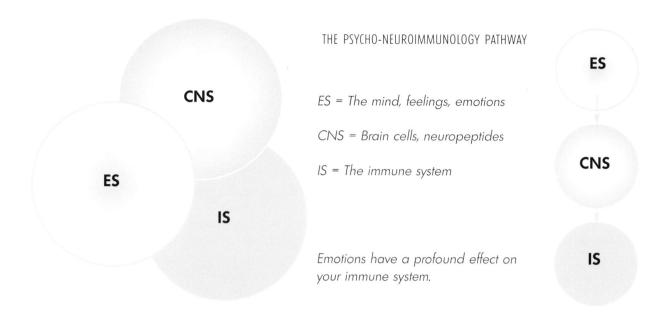

THE PSYCHO-NEUROIMMUNOLOGY PATHWAY

ES = The mind, feelings, emotions

CNS = Brain cells, neuropeptides

IS = The immune system

Emotions have a profound effect on your immune system.

PSYCHO-NEUROIMMUNOLOGY

'The mind has a great influence over the body and maladies often have their origin there.'
Molière

Psycho-neuroimmunology (PNI) is the scientific study of mind-body activity, where thoughts and emotions are linked with physical responses and the immune system. This occurs through a pathway that links the pituitary gland and the hypothalamus (both parts of your brain) with the adrenal glands, which release stress hormones.

Your emotions result in the release of neuro-peptides, or neurotransmitters, which travel across the dendrites connecting your brain cells. These neuropeptides then attach themselves to receptor sites on your immune cells. In this way, feelings of happiness and joy can boost your immune system, whereas the toxic emotions – anxiety, depression, pessimism, sadness and negativity – have the opposite effect of depressing the immune system.

It is clear that mind-body exercises, as well as mind-body therapies, play an important part in promoting a feeling of wellbeing, quieting the mind and creating tranquillity as an antidote to stress and negative emotions. Even for those people who are coping well with their everyday lives, mind-body exercise is a way to enhance memory and maintain optimum brain function.

One of the most effective ways of dealing with toxic emotions is to practise laughter therapy. It is difficult to cultivate a sense of humour if you do not have one, but you can make an effort to incorporate laughter into your life.
- Read the comics in your local newspaper.
- Watch old comedy movies.
- Find a book of jokes or humorous quotations.
- Join a laughter club. They really do exist! A medical doctor in Mumbai (Bombay) started India's first laughter club and there are now several hundred in the country. You could even start your own.

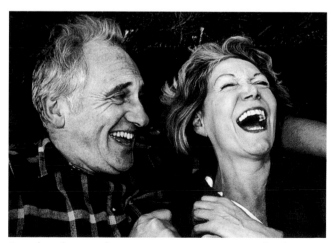

Laughter boosts the immune system, aerates the lungs, improves circulation and lubricates the soul.

PROTECT YOUR MEMORY

There is no need to get upset if you cannot remember where you have put your house keys – you should worry only if you cannot remember what they are for. Virtually everyone has memory lapses from time to time. You bump into an old friend at a party, but cannot remember his name. Are you worried you are heading for Alzheimer's disease? You should not be concerned unless memory impairment becomes a frequent occurrence.

Why does memory decline with age?

- Age-associated memory impairment (AAMI) occurs when the flow of traffic, or conductivity, of our brain cells slows down.
- Poor diet, lack of exercise, too much alcohol, low energy levels and an overall poor health cause deterioration in all our brain functions, including in the memory.
- Stress has an adverse effect on memory.
- Free radicals result in the equivalent of rusting, destroying brain cell connections. They also lead to atherosclerosis, or fatty deposits within the

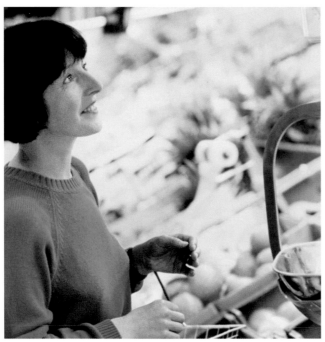

Test and challenge your memory by visiting the super-market without a shopping list.

blood vessels, interrupting blood flow to the brain. People with high blood pressure generally have lower scores on tests for memory than people with normal blood pressure.

- Distraction is more of a problem with ageing. You may take your car to fill up with petrol, then go into a shop and wonder what you went there for. Information can slip out of your working memory before you have a chance to store it, so it is important to concentrate on one task at a time. This is in contrast to younger adults who have the ability to 'multitask' – they may, for instance, be able to read the newspaper at the same time as listening to the news on the radio.
- Medication overload can be partly responsible. Many older people may be taking sleeping pills, blood pressure pills or analgesics. The effect of these may produce impaired clarity of thought and memory impairment.

How can you improve memory?

- Follow a diet rich in antioxidants, especially vitamins C, E and betacarotene. Researchers suggest that vitamin E is a weapon against Alzheimer's disease. Further studies show an 80 per cent lower risk for vascular dementia in people consuming adequate amounts of vitamins E and C. Other research has promoted the intake of the B group of vitamins. Vitamin B12 is often deficient in older people, and supplements greatly improve memory.
- Physical exercise increases blood flow to the brain. Walking for 30 minutes every day will improve your memory and all mental functions.
- Mental exercise is equally important. The brain responds to stimulation, with improved circulation nourishing and strengthening nerve cells. Good mental workouts include: scrabble, bridge, crossword puzzles, learning a new language, learning computer skills and reading thought-provoking books.
- Review your medications with your doctor.
- Avoid distractions as inattention is a primary cause of forgetting. Absentmindednesss is often associated with older people, but is really a form of inattention. You may forget where you parked your car if you do not pay enough attention when you are

parking it. The basic skill of successful memory is to focus and concentrate on the present moment.

- Hormone replacement with oestrogens, testosterone or pregnenalone can be discussed with your doctor.

Alzheimer's disease (AD)

This progressive, neurodegenerative disorder is probably the most feared disease of ageing men and women. Some 20 per cent of people over 65 and 50 per cent of those over 85 have AD.

To date, no definite cause has been found, although risk factors include advancing age, a family history of Alzheimer's, and a specific gene known as Apo E4. Multiple factors are thought to be involved. Diagnosis is made on the history and symptoms, as well as new imaging techniques. The brains of Alzheimer's patients contain decreased amounts of the enzyme needed to make the neurotransmitter, acetylcholine. In addition, changes in the brain include the formation of clumps of dead cells known as 'plaques' and abnormal fibres called 'tangles'.

Can you prevent AD? Since there is as yet no concrete evidence about its cause, you can only adopt

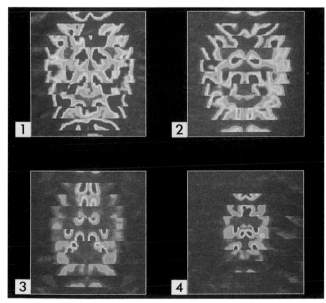

MRI scans of the brain.
1. Healthy brain. 2. Early Alzheimer's disease.
3. Late Alzheimer's disease. 4. Infant's brain.

THE DEGENERATION OF THE BRAIN CELL/ALZHEIMER'S

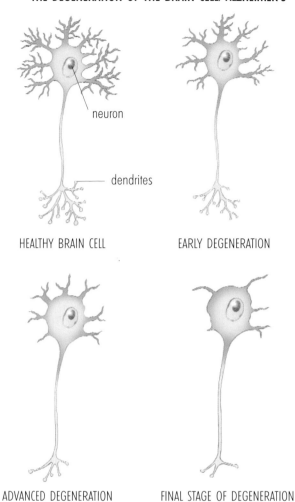

HEALTHY BRAIN CELL   EARLY DEGENERATION

ADVANCED DEGENERATION   FINAL STAGE OF DEGENERATION

Above: The healthy brain cell has numerous dendrites connecting it to other brain cells. As deterioration occurs, dendrites are gradually lost, resulting in minimal connections between cells or neurons.

the preventive measures recommended in this chapter. In other words, feed your brain with the correct nutrients, exercise it both physically and mentally, and try to avoid excitotoxins and other potential toxins. In addition, taking antioxidants, especially vitamins E, C and alpha lipoic acid, can be recommended. If AD has been diagnosed, there are a number of experimental drugs currently being prescribed and new ones in development.

It may not be Alzheimer's

Other causes of memory loss must be distinguished from AD. Age-associated memory impairment (AAMI), for instance, affects men and women over the age of 50, with gradual memory loss over a period of years while intellectual function remains normal.

Vascular dementia is caused by a series of small strokes with similar symptoms to AD, while over-medication is an important preventable cause of memory impairment and mental confusion. Your ability to metabolize medications declines as you age, so smaller doses of medication should be given to older people. The liver's ability to detoxify drugs is also diminished, so the levels of these rise in the bloodstream. Common culprits include sleeping pills, tranquillizers, painkillers and blood pressure pills.

Memory loss in older people

- Alzheimer's disease
- Age-associated memory impairment
- Mini strokes
- Overmedication
- Nutrient deficiencies
- Excessive alcohol
- Disuse

BALANCING YOUR BRAIN

Right- and left-brain integration is important. To understand or make jokes, for instance, you need both sides of your brain. If you are irritable, anxious or depressed, this can usually be remedied by implementing some left-brain activity.

Many people are left-brain dominant. In order to create balance between the two hemispheres, you can practise some of these right-brain activities.

- Listen to music, specifically impressionistic compositions, New Age, Debussy, pan pipes.
- Take up painting or visit art galleries.
- Pursue creative hobbies.
- Appreciate the beauties of nature.

In his book, *Use Both Sides of your Brain*, psychologist Tony Buzan introduces us to the concept of 'mind mapping'. An internationally recognized teacher of memory training and study techniques, he shows how you can improve memory, creative thinking and problem solving while integrating both right and left sides of the brain. Instead of the conventional method of making notes by writing at the top and working down in sentences or lists, he advises that you should start with a central idea and branch out with satellite ideas following a general theme. In this way, the most important points are in the middle, and the connections and links are visible. Equally importantly, the task of keeping notes, making speeches or solving problems encourages creative right-brain thinking.

YOUR LEFT BRAIN	YOUR RIGHT BRAIN
Logical	Intuitive
Makes lists	Creative
Numbers	Visual, sees the overall picture
Analytical	Uses imagination
Follows orderly sequences	Abstract
Successful	Empathetic
Materialistic	Enjoys music, rhythm, colour
Unfeeling	Emotional

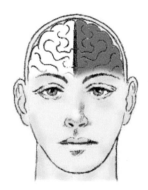 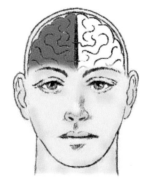

LEFT BRAIN   **RIGHT BRAIN**

Left-brain dominant people are analytical and logical; right-brain dominant people are creative, visual and emotional.

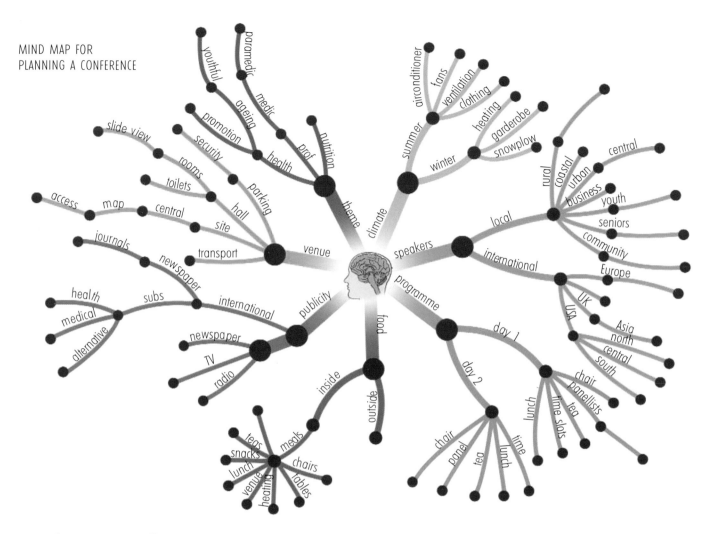

A mind map is an excellent way to solve problems, think creatively and work towards improving your memory.

Are male and female brains different?

The *corpus callosum* is a mass of fibres connecting the left and right sides of the brain. In women these connecting fibres are more diffuse, allowing free flow of information between both sides. In men there are fewer fibres, resulting in the compartmentalization of right- and left-brain functions. Men can perform two different activities at once – for example, talking while reverse parking a car. This may be difficult for a woman because the two activities will interfere with each other.

In women, emotions are held in both sides of the brain. A man keeps his emotions locked up in his right brain, while the ability to express his feelings in speech lies on the left side. If a man experiences

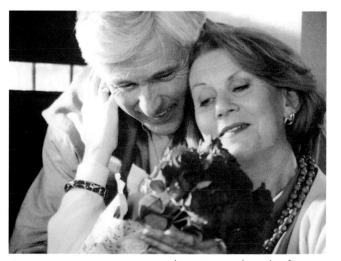

A man may express emotion by giving a bunch of roses.

the feeling of love (in his right brain) he may find it difficult to access the verbal left brain to say, 'I love you'. He may go out and buy a bunch of roses instead. Women, with their free flow of information between both sides of the brain, have better capabilities of intuitive understanding and the ability to communicate their emotions.

What happens as male and female brains age?

Male brains are larger than female brains, but they age more quickly, with shrinkage and loss of volume as shown by MRI techniques.

Male brains secrete more serotonin than female brains, which may be one of the reasons why females have a higher incidence of depression and eating disorders.

Hormones have a major effect on brain functioning. The male hormone, testosterone, increases aggressive behaviour, competitiveness, assertiveness and independence, while the female hormone, oestrogen, has the opposite effect. In keeping with the concept of men 'mellowing' with age, the male desire for dominance fades gradually after the age of about 55 with the andropause, making men less assertive and aggressive. They begin to enjoy smelling the roses and may even start washing the dishes. When women's oestrogen levels decrease during the menopause, they may become crotchety and more assertive due to the unopposed small levels of testosterone.

Thus as men and women age, their behaviour becomes similar as a result of each sex's individual waning hormones.

BRAIN GYM

Brain Gym is a series of simple, effective exercises to improve and maintain the brain's fitness. Developed by American teacher Paul Dennison to help children with learning problems, it has also helped older people to improve brain integration by fine-tuning eye-hand co-ordination, memory and concentration. People suffering from anxiety, depression and chronic stress have improved after two months of doing these exercises for 15 minutes every day. Brain Gym is not a magical remedy, but it has a scientific neurophysiological basis.

These simple exercises are ideal for older people and take only a few minutes of your time every day. You can do them while you are waiting for a phone call, in the bedroom, in the garden, or in your office. You can do them sitting down or standing.

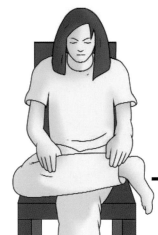

FOOT FLEX
Sit up straight, resting the right ankle on the left knee. Hold your calf muscle between your thumbs and fingers, massaging it towards the knee with one hand and towards the ankle with the other. Alternately flex and point your foot while you massage the muscle. Repeat with the other leg.

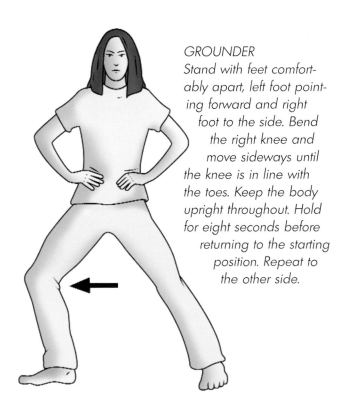

GROUNDER
Stand with feet comfortably apart, left foot pointing forward and right foot to the side. Bend the right knee and move sideways until the knee is in line with the toes. Keep the body upright throughout. Hold for eight seconds before returning to the starting position. Repeat to the other side.

What are the benefits?

- Brain gym enhances communication between left and right brain.
- It improves blood circulation to brain cells.
- It activates neurotransmitters, sending messages across the dendrites between brain cells.
- It improves memory and concentration.
- It is an antidote for stress and anxiety.

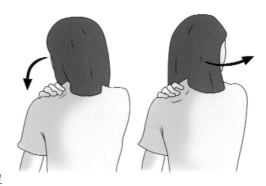

OWL
Sit straight. Massage the large shoulder muscle that runs from your neck to your shoulder. Turn your head to look over your left shoulder, then over your right shoulder, saying 'mmm' as you turn your head. Repeat on the other side.

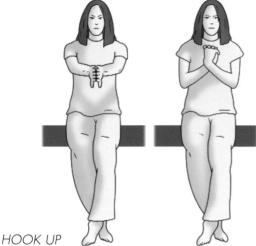

HOOK UP
Sit with ankles crossed. Stretch arms in front of you, backs of your hands together and thumbs facing down. Cross your hands at the wrists so the palms are together and interlace your fingers. Bend hands down and inwards towards your chest. Relax the shoulders and put your tongue against the highest part of your palate. Breathe slowly and deeply several times.

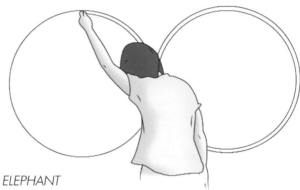

ELEPHANT
Stand up straight with left arm stretched out and pressed against your ear, eyes focused on your finger-tips and beyond. Moving from your midline, make a large circle anticlockwise to the left, then clockwise to the right. Repeat with the other arm.

POSITIVE POINTS
The positive points are halfway between your eyebrows and hairline, directly above the pupils of your eyes as you look forward. Stimulate these points with both hands or with the thumb and index finger of one hand.

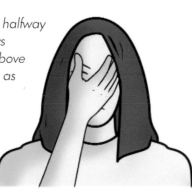

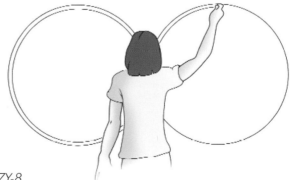

LAZY-8
Stand up straight, holding your right thumb out in front of you at eye level. Watch your thumb as you move it a few times in a large circle to the left, then to the right. Repeat with your left thumb.

MUSIC AND THE BRAIN

'Music hath charms to soothe the savage breast,
To soften rocks, or bend a knotted oak.'
William Congreve

Most of us enjoy listening to music without analyzing the effect it has on us. We may feel stimulated after listening to a stirring Beethoven symphony, calm and serene after hearing a Baroque fugue, uplifted after a Gregorian chant, agitated after a Stravinsky composition, disturbed after rock and rap, or relaxed after floating through pan pipes and flute music.

However we respond, music produces both mental and physical effects. It has a definite effect on brain functioning. A Japanese study of patients undergoing music therapy found that after an hour there was a dramatic increase in natural killer (NK) cells in the blood, indicating an improved immune response. NK cells are white blood cells produced by the thymus gland as part of the body's natural defence system.

Another study in the United States looked at the effects of drumming on the immune system. The group of drummers studied was found to have more NK cells, increased DHEA levels and reduced cortisol levels. Researchers concluded that drumming has the potential to combat stress.

How effective is Mozart?

In his book, *The Mozart Effect*, classically trained musician Don Campbell writes about the power of music to strengthen the mind. He has researched techniques to help people to learn more effectively, and ways to improve mood and mental functioning.

Does the Mozart effect really exist? Researchers have found that listening to Mozart's sonata in D major for two pianos (K448) can improve reasoning skills in human subjects. The experiment was taken further in animal studies when a group of rats was exposed to this sonata for 60 days. As controls, other rats were exposed to modern rock music or silence. They were then tested for their ability to negotiate a maze. The Mozart group completed the maze significantly more quickly and with fewer errors.

Mozart's piano concerto number 23 in A major (K488) has also proved to be effective in improving clarity of thought, concentration and memory.

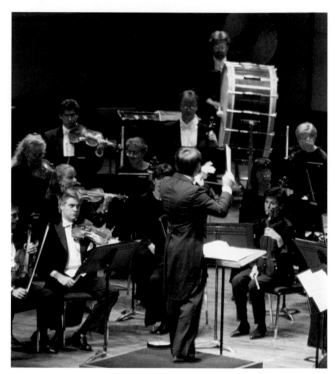

Listening to music lowers your stress cortisol levels and balances the right and left brain.

How does music affect the brain?

The 19th century philosopher, Friedrich Nietzsche, said: 'Without music life would be a mistake.' Certainly, music is one of the most enriching and enjoyable ways of improving your brain's functions.

1. Music can slow down and balance brain waves. During your daily activities, as well as when you experience negative emotions, the electroencephalograph (EEG) used to measure brain waves will pick up beta waves. When you are calm, alert and centred, you generate alpha waves. During meditation, and when you practise Tai Chi or Qi Gong, you display theta waves. It has been found that music of 60 beats per minute can move brain waves from beta to the alpha range, thereby increasing alertness and wellbeing.

2. Listening to music can lower stress levels by decreasing output of cortisol. Try listening to a Chopin nocturne.

3. Music has the ability to lower blood pressure and reduce muscle tension.

4. It can boost the immune system, e.g. the effect of drumming.

5. It can increase the release of beta-endorphins (happiness hormones). Music that has an emotional impact – religious music, marching bands and soundtracks from some movies – will evoke a feeling of joyous upliftment. Mahler's symphony number 2 in C minor ('Resurrection') ends with overwhelming emotion, leaving the listener with a feeling of profound spiritual wellbeing.

THINK YOUTHFULLY

The brain of a child is curious and full of wonderment at the new and joyful experiences encountered each day. Children are full of enthusiasm. At least part of the secret of youthful ageing is to retain this enthusiasm as you grow older.

American industrialist, Henry Ford, is said to have commented: 'You can do anything if you have enthusiasm. Enthusiasm is the yeast that makes your hopes rise to the stars. Enthusiasm is the sparkle in your eyes, the swing in your gait, the grip of your hand, the irresistible surge of energy to execute your ideas. Enthusiasts are fighters. They have staying qualities. With enthusiasm there is accomplishment. Without it, there are only alibis.'

Your youthful brain is enthusiastic, playful, flexible, relaxed, creative, adaptable and adventurous. Your brain will thrive on new experiences and new knowledge. Try to read at least one book a week, including classics and current fiction, as well as spiritual and self-help literature. Aim to learn something new every day. Stimulate those neurons and visualize your dendrites sprouting new tentacles.

Here is what an 85-year-old with a sense of humour, had to say about staying young at heart:
'If I had my life over, I would take more chances, I would eat more ice cream and less beans. I have been one of those persons who never goes anywhere without a thermometer, a hot water bottle, a raincoat and a parachute. If I had to do it again, I would travel lighter, I would go to more dances, I would ride more merry-go-rounds, I would pick more daisies.'

ACTION PLAN

➤ Feed your brain with brain-boosting nutrients, avoid bad fats and keep blood sugar levels stable.

➤ Start taking brain-enhancing supplements, especially vitamins C and E.

➤ Exercise your brain mentally and physically.

➤ Create balance by incorporating right-brain activities into your daily life.

➤ Take time each day to meditate, relax, and listen to music.

➤ Drink six to eight glasses of water daily to keep your brain well hydrated.

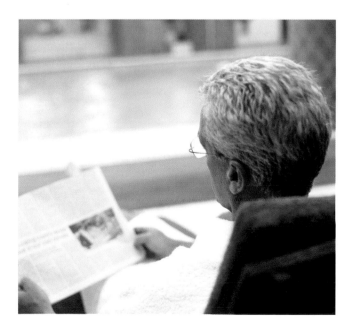

Left: Reading stimulates brain cells to form new dendrites.

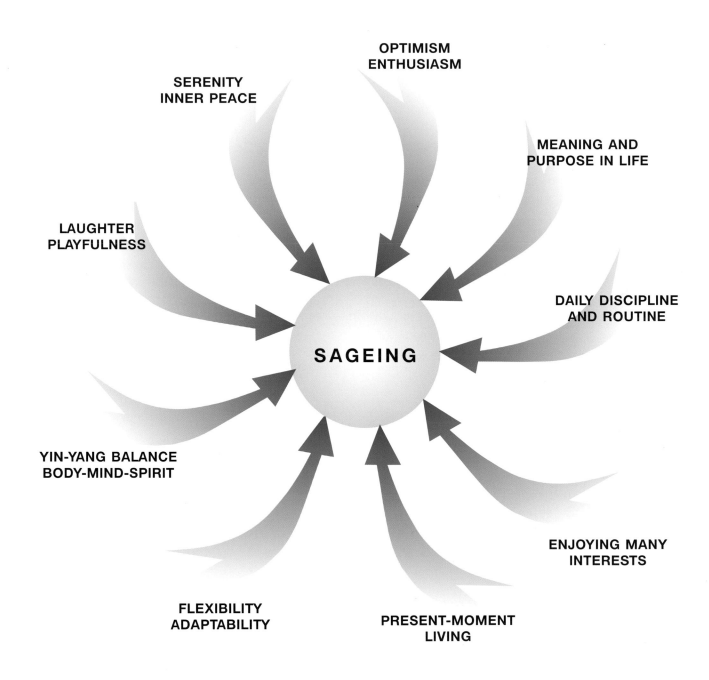

SAGEING AND SPIRITUAL AGEING

'Life is either an incredible adventure or it is nothing at all.' **Helen Keller**

By definition, a sage is a person who has acquired wisdom. This may be one of the most valuable benefits of growing older. We learn to tame the passions of youth. While gathering knowledge and experience along the way – often rocky and sometimes painful – we are able to acquire a global perspective of life's events.

There have been many definitions of the ages of man (and woman), some of them flippant and others more profound. Actress and bawdy performer, Sophie Tucker, jokingly remarked: 'Under the age of 18 a girl needs good parents. From 18 to 35 she needs good looks. From 35 to 55 she needs a good personality, and thereafter she needs a good share portfolio.'

In more serious vein, the Talmud describes the ages of man as follows:

- 40 years is the age for understanding
- 50 years is the age for giving advice
- 60 years is the age for acquiring wisdom
- 70 years is the age for growing white hair
- 80 years is the age for the special strength of age

Thus, according to the Talmud, we should become sages at the age of 60, which coincides with the concept of 'late adulthood' as described by Daniel Levinson in his book, *The Seasons of a Man's Life*. Levinson and co-workers at Yale University in the United States conducted extensive psychosocial studies of adult development throughout the life cycle.

Levinson refers to the study of adult development that was initially commenced by pioneering psychoanalyst, Sigmund Freud, and continued by Carl Jung. As part of normal development, Jung regarded the young adult to be involved with the demands of work and family while still attached to the emotional conflicts of childhood. He found that the age of 40 was the 'noon of life' and a time for significant change. Levinson went on to describe the phases of a person's life cycle as 'seasons'. He regarded the age of 40 to 45 as the mid-life transition, and 45 to 60 as middle adulthood, with 60 as the starting point for the period of late adulthood.

Describing the over-sixties as men and women who have entered the period of late adulthood would certainly seem to be more acceptable than the often-used terms 'elderly' and 'senior citizen', which have negative connotations.

For those who have held positions of authority and power in the corporate world, it can be traumatic to move from centre-stage, to retire and become 'wet leaves'. This is a term used by some Japanese women to describe their husbands after retirement. Wet leaves because the husbands stick around all day and they cannot get rid of them; wet leaves because they never found time to develop hobbies and interests outside the workplace.

Many senior business executives do become depressed after retirement. At the age of 60 or 65, depression may be due to other causes such as hormonal decline, known as the andropause (*see* pages 56–57), but a blood test to estimate testosterone levels will pick this up. Retirement should not be a period of decline, but one of development and new opportunities.

The age after retirement is often described as the 'third age'. A better description would be to call it the 'age of living'. This is the period of your life when you generally have the freedom to travel, explore, expand your

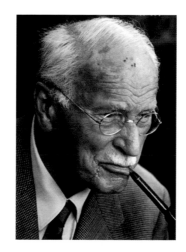

Carl Jung

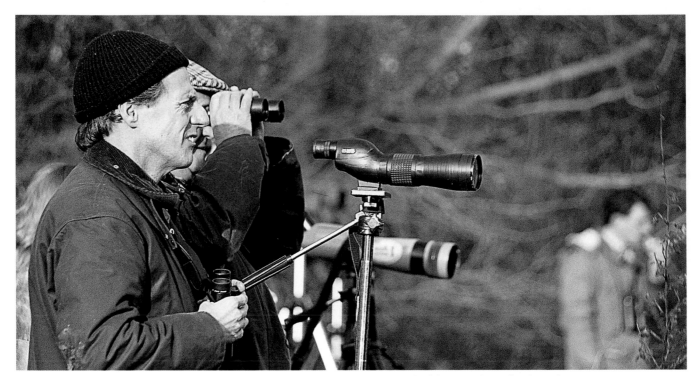

The 'age of living' is a time during which you should be able to enjoy hobbies such as birdwatching.

hobbies, improve your computer skills, learn to tango, volunteer for community projects, be a mentor and spend time with your grandchildren. For you to enjoy this time to the full, it is essential for you to be healthy and well. You should not enter the 'age of living' with painful arthritic joints, high blood pressure or a failing memory. You need to maintain the vibrancy and enthusiasm of your youth and your spirit of adventure – but with the wisdom that you have acquired from years of experience.

There is no quick fix or magic anti-ageing potion that will make you younger. Cosmetic surgery, botox injections and liposuction may make your face and body look more youthful, but they will not prevent chronic degenerative problems such as arthritis, diabetes or heart disease. Nor will they prevent you from possibly needing a hip replacement, bypass surgery, or long-term chronic medication. You may even decide to follow a popular rapid weight-loss diet, but this will result in loss of lean tissue and muscle, with subsequent weight gain and additional fat gain once you resume normal eating. The simple truth is that there is no alternative to the often-difficult task of changing your lifestyle.

Several studies involving healthy centenarians have been conducted. Perhaps the New England Centenarian study in the United States is one of the most comprehensive. Started in 1999, it was implemented by researchers at Harvard University. This ongoing study has so far identified certain characteristics that appear to be prevalent in centenarians. They eat and drink in moderation, stay in touch with their friends and family, and keep their brains active with a variety of activities and projects. In general, they score low on tests for negative or toxic emotions such as anxiety, hostility and depression, but are collectively more relaxed and stress resistant than the average population.

Other studies of centenarians have found a number of additional qualities.

CENTENARIAN QUALITIES
• Live in the present moment; do not live in the past or for the future.
• Never procrastinate – be proactive.
• Never functionally retire: continue to learn and grow, explore new horizons, accept challenges and new experiences.

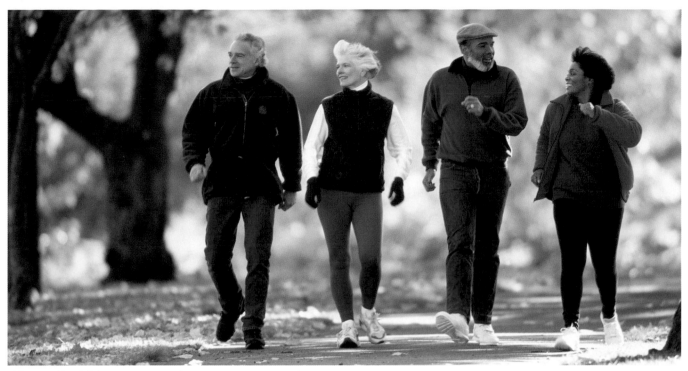

Above: Youthful agers are enthusiastic, positive and optimistic people who generally also have plenty of vitality and joie de vivre.
Below right: Painting is a creative right-brain activity.

- Maintain a meaning and purpose in life: everyone has some unique ability or talent that he or she can implement.
- Remain optimistic, with a positive outlook on life.
- Keep discipline in your life: organize your days, exercise, meditate, relax, eat enough fruit and vegetables.
- Be interested in many different things rather than occupied with just one interest. Have a variety of hobbies, sports and activities.
- Grow older with a sense of humour, playfulness, laughter and spontaneity.
- Cultivate inner peace, serenity and tranquillity. Take time to be alone and relax, listen to music and enjoy nature.
- Be adaptable and flexible enough to accept change. Change is inevitable and you need to accept this and 'go with the flow'. The fact is that you will become old if you believe that things cannot or should not be changed.

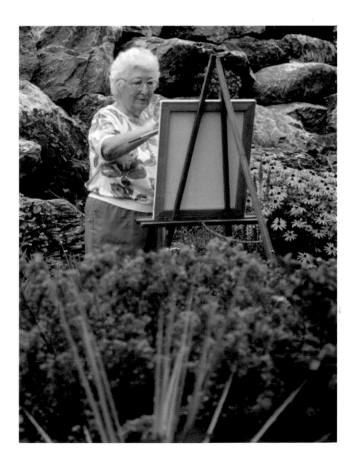

In earlier times, human life expectancy was much less than it is today. This was largely due to the impact of disease, lack of hygiene and a high infant mortality. During the time of the Roman Empire, for instance, average life expectancy was less than 30 years, while in the 15th and 16th centuries it was certainly no more than 40.

It is therefore remarkable to read essays written by an Italian aristocrat, Luigi Cornaro, who was born in Venice in 1467 and died in 1565 – aged 98. After an early life filled with overindulgence of every kind, Cornaro resolved to change his ways. His first essay,

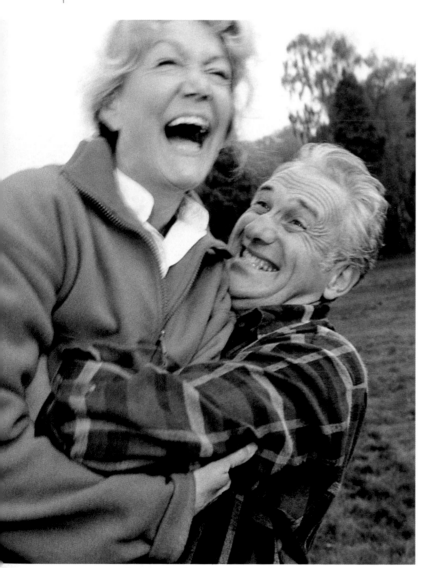

Laughter is the best medicine.

written at the age of 83, described how to achieve health and longevity by reducing calorie intake – 'constantly rising from the table with a disposition to eat and drink still more'. He curtailed his intake to a strict 350g (12oz) of food each day. For relaxation he rode his horse, 'mounting without assistance', spent time in his garden, read good books, and spent time with his friends, whom he considered 'valuable for their good sense and manners'. He journeyed to neighbouring cities to see palaces, gardens and antiquities, and played and sang with his grandchildren. He wrote another essay at the age of 95, proclaiming that he was still enjoying 'conversing with men of bright parts and superior understanding' and that 'without the least fatigue' he was 'able to study the most difficult subjects'. Luigi Cornaro was an excellent example of the best centenarian qualities.

THOUGHTS CAN MAKE YOU YOUNG

The old saying, 'You are over the hill at 50,' does not apply today. You can be old at 50 and youthful at 80. There are many people of 70 or 80 years old who look and act at least 15 to 20 years younger because they think youthfully. In fact, it is possible for you to grow younger by changing your thoughts. Ignore the date on your birth certificate and visualize each part of your body as it was in its prime. Attend to your posture and put a spring into your step. With regular exercise, daily stretching and correct nutrition, you should suffer no pain or stiffness.

Linked to your thoughts, your feelings can either make you old before your time or they can help you to achieve a high level of wellness. Anxiety, tension, anger and depression, as well as fear, guilt and pessimism, are all toxic emotions to be avoided. By contrast, joy, happiness, enthusiasm and optimism are anti-ageing qualities well worth striving for.

LAUGHTER

'Angels can fly because they take themselves lightly.' G.K. Chesterton

When we are children, we are able to laugh easily and be playful. As we grow into adulthood many of us lose the ability to laugh, to have a sense of humour, and 'to take ourselves lightly'.

What has laughter to do with turning back the ageing clock? In his book, *Anatomy of an Illness*, Norman Cousins tells how he was cured of a potentially fatal illness by watching comedy movies. He used laughter as therapy and, in fact, laughter is truly an excellent medicine. It is impossible to feel sad when you are laughing: the toxic emotions of anxiety, tension, anger and depression simply drain away.

Scientific studies have shown that laughter stimulates the immune system, increasing the number of your natural killer cells, which are the particular white blood cells that are involved in fighting bacteria, viruses and even cancer cells.

Do you lack a sense of humour? It is an interesting fact that although most individuals can admit to a variety of negative traits, they will rarely admit to a lack of a sense of humour. Learn to laugh more frequently. Begin with reading jokes and comics, play with a puppy or a kitten, and play with your grandchildren. If all else fails, join a laughter club (*see* page 101).

THE YIN-YANG PRINCIPLE

Why have Eastern therapies and exercises such as Tai Chi, yoga, shiatsu and acupressure been included in this book? It is because Chinese medicine, in particular, focuses on the underlying causes of disease, contrasting with Western medicine, which treats symptoms by 'killing the messenger'. Chinese therapies concentrate on strengthening the immune system, as well as activating the body's energy pathways. Their medical system, based on the belief that disease and ill health are due to an imbalance of body functions or emotions, has been tested and practised for over 3000 years.

The terms 'yin' and 'yang' express opposing forces. Various therapies, physical exercise, acupuncture, acupressure and herbs are used to create balance and harmony, as well as to activate a person's basic energy levels. As opposite, alternating forces, yin and yang have to interact and achieve balance. It is for the individual to find this balance – something that requires adaptation and adjustment to every situation and relationship in life. You need to strive to achieve balance and harmony both in yourself and in your environment.

In Chinese medicine the concepts of yin and yang have been given attributes such as female and male, coldness and heat, dark and light. The therapy aims to create a balance, for example, you might be diagnosed as having an excess of yin, or a deficiency of yang, which needs to be brought into balance.

YIN	YANG
Female, passive	Male, active
Coldness	Heat
Dark	Strength
Weakness	Light
Contraction	Expansion
Interior	Exterior
Below	Above

Below: The symbol for yin and yang, embodying balance.

You can apply the yin-yang principle to the process of ageing youthfully. By creating harmony between yin and yang you can balance mind, body and spirit. This creates a healthy environment, facilitating your path to optimum health.

In simple terms, when your life is out of balance you become vulnerable to a variety of illnesses. A common example is the business executive who is a workaholic, has no time for exercise, eats fast foods, drinks coffee all day and relaxes at night with alcohol. He is an excellent candidate for a heart attack.

It is a good idea to examine your own life. Are you devoting enough time to your friends, family and recreation? Social connectedness counteracts the harmful effects of the stress hormone, cortisol. On the other hand, loneliness is a predictor of premature death. Do you take time each day to exercise? Do you spend some quiet time alone each day? Are you mindful of the quality and quantity of food that you eat? Is your life in balance?

IS YOUR LIFE IN BALANCE?

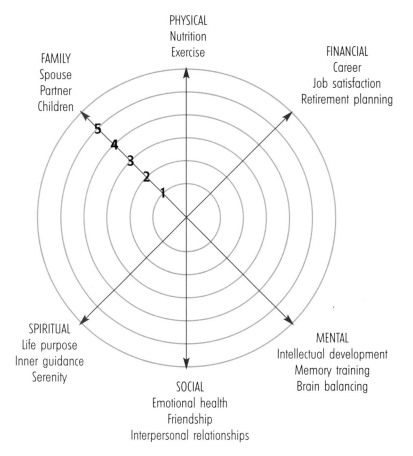

On a scale of 1 to 5, estimate whether you are devoting attention to all areas of your life

PHYSICAL
Nutrition
Exercise

FINANCIAL
Career
Job satisfaction
Retirement planning

FAMILY
Spouse
Partner
Children

MENTAL
Intellectual development
Memory training
Brain balancing

SPIRITUAL
Life purpose
Inner guidance
Serenity

SOCIAL
Emotional health
Friendship
Interpersonal relationships

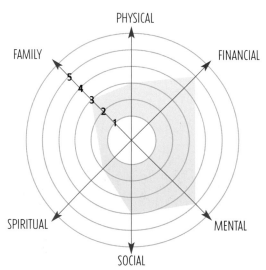

EXAMPLE: The unbalanced wheel of a 50-year-old businessman, financially successful, who spends considerable time away from home.

CHOICES

'If you have not the strength to impose your own terms upon life, you must accept the terms it offers you.' **T.S. Eliot**

Only 20 per cent of your life expectancy is, in fact, determined by your genes. The rest depends on your environment and on personal choices as to how you wish to live your life.

There is a well-known saying that you are what you eat, and it is true that the food and drink you consume either nourishes or damages the trillions of cells in your body. Food can either enhance your energy or sap it. It is estimated that the DNA in your cells is subjected to about 10,000 free radical hits per day, which would cause considerable damage and premature ageing if not counterbalanced by a

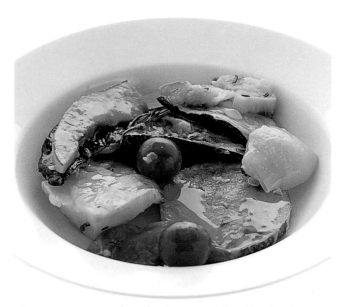

Create energy and vitality by eating healthy foods.

hefty dose of antioxidants. Exciting new research has revealed that certain nutrients in foods, the nutriceuticals (which are powerful antioxidants), can fight free radicals, and thus help to slow down or prevent cellular ageing.

A plant requires a variety of minerals in order to flourish and grow. Lack of magnesium in the soil will reveal itself by causing yellowing of the leaves. If your body lacks magnesium, which is the case with many people, are you taking note of the signals of magnesium deficiency? Your body requires an optimum variety of vitamins and minerals to function in a youthful way. Are you overloading yourself with wheat, sugar or dairy products? Are you experiencing digestive problems or stiff and aching joints? By regular detoxing and by reducing or even eliminating these foods, you may experience a dramatic improvement in your health. Scientific studies have indicated that a diet of more fruit and vegetables and less fat is associated with a reduced risk of Alzheimer's disease. So it appears that what is good for the heart is good for the brain too.

Looking at the long-lived populations in the world we see that the Japanese, particularly the Okinawans, consume a diet that is low in sugars and fats, but rich in vegetables, soya products and fish.

The Mediterranean diet, which is also associated with a lower risk of heart disease and increased longevity, is rich in vegetables and olive oil.

You have now been presented with evidence that certain foods will prevent degenerative disease and improve your healthspan. The choice is yours as to whether you are likely either to suffer ill health or enjoy vibrant good health.

Remember that as you age, you need to reduce your calorie intake. Visualize the amount of food that you can hold in your outstretched palms, which is about the size of your stomach. Practise what the Okinawans call 'hara hachi bu' and only eat until you are 80 per cent full, no more.

Animal research has shown that not only do calorie-restricted rats and mice live longer, they look and act younger, they are more active, they keep their fur, and they are less likely to develop cancer and degenerative diseases.

In 1991, gerontologist Roy Walford spent two years in the Biosphere 2 greenhouse in the Arizona desert. On a calorie-restricted diet consisting mainly of vegetables, legumes, grains and fruit, the participants experienced improvements in their cholesterol levels, blood pressure and glucose metabolism.

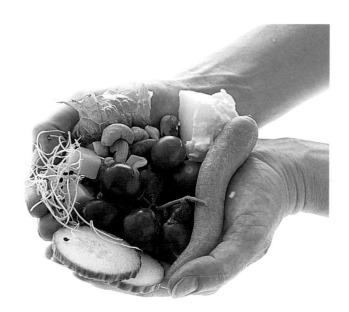

Calorie restriction extends the lifespan. Eat no more than will fit into your cupped palms.

The other important choice you have to make is one regarding exercise. Regular exercise can turn back the ageing clock by some 10 to 15 years. Our bodies were designed for action. No matter what your age, you can start an exercise programme that will increase your muscular strength, improve your balance and flexibility, increase your energy levels and strengthen your bones. The choice is yours.

So, too, can you choose to keep your brain vibrant and to remain actively engaged in life. You can choose to adopt centenarian qualities. You can ensure that you breathe clean air and drink pure water. You can avoid premature ageing caused by taking numerous unnecessary medications, known as 'polypharmacy'. You can choose to be helpless or you can achieve control of your life. All these choices can have either a positive or negative outcome; they can be either ageing or anti-ageing.

With the mapping of the human genome, stem cell research, telomerase therapy, tissue engineering and cloning, we may one day be able to engineer new organs, repair failing organs and extend life to a possible 120 years. A bioengineered kidney may replace dialysis, a new liver may replace one that is damaged by hepatitis or cirrhosis, and a fresh pancreas may bring relief to insulin-dependent diabetics. In addition, quadriplegics may even be able to walk after new cells are grown in damaged spinal cords. However, all these developments have serious ethical implications, apart from technical and economic considerations.

Instead of hoping for increased life expectancy, it is more important for us to concentrate on increasing health expectancy by making appropriate lifestyle choices. Most of us can count on living to 85, but our lifestyle choices can either eliminate or exaggerate chronic illnesses that make the senior years so disabling for many people.

SPIRITUAL AGEING

'For this is a journey that men make; to find themselves.
If they fail in this, it doesn't matter much what else they find.' **James Michener**

As we grow older we need to accept the choices we have made in earlier years, without regret. Every circumstance has a purpose and helps us to grow. We need to live in the present, with no regrets about the past or worries about the future.

When we talk of spiritual ageing we are not talking about religion. Spirituality is in essence the individual experience of getting in touch with your internal guidance and higher self.

This is the time for you to develop a new way of thinking. If the changes need to be radical, it will require a paradigm shift. If you are already on the right track, then perhaps all you will need is some fine-tuning. This is your journey towards ageing youthfully. You will take personal responsibility for your health and wellbeing. You will listen to your body, to your feelings and to your intuition.

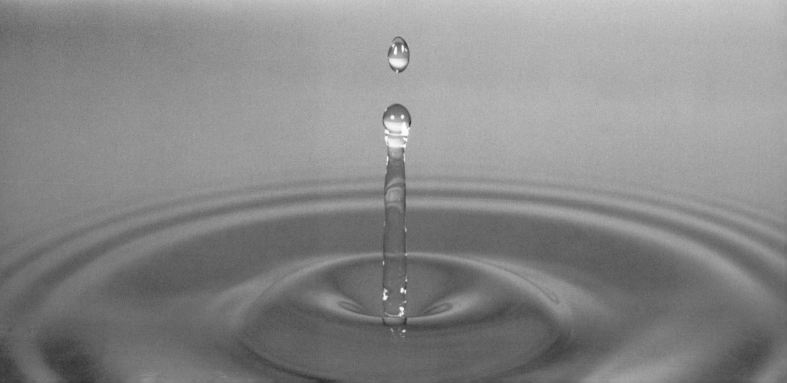

With spiritual ageing we become aware of, and receptive to, the concept of synchronicity. This term was first used by psychiatrist Carl Jung to describe a 'meaningful coincidence'. For example, we may require some particular information, and then soon afterwards we encounter someone who provides us with exactly what we need. Synchronicity may act as a helper in some small task or it may lead to a major shift in life direction.

What about inner guidance and intuition? Do you think you are intuitive? Of course you are. The problem is that many people tend to ignore their inner voice. Intuition is an inner 'knowing' that emerges from your subconscious mind. The sensation of 'knowing' is directed towards a future event, and you are able to make decisions based on a gut feeling rather than rational data.

Recognizing and utilizing intuition and synchronicities is an exciting way to enhance purpose and meaning in your life. In his book, *Man's Search for Meaning*, psychiatrist Victor Frankl, himself a Holocaust survivor, described how prisoners in concentration camps during World War II managed to survive because of their incredibly strong will and belief in there being a purpose for living. We all need to maintain our purpose for living; the alternative is depression and bodily decline.

With spiritual ageing you should be able to dissolve negative feelings of guilt, fear, jealousy and resentment and replace them with feelings of serenity, forgiveness, gratitude and unconditional loving. You can achieve serenity and equanimity by spending a quiet time alone every day, learning to quieten the mind. Instead of 'awfulizing' as you grow older, you need to be consciously grateful for your family and friends, for your health, for your attributes, and for all the good things in your life. It may help you to start a 'gratitude journal' and to write down a few things that you are grateful for every day.

The period of late adulthood will be a rich and rewarding time of your life if you forget about the terms 'old age', 'senior citizen' and 'elderly'. Focus instead on remaining youthful during what can be better termed the 'age of living'.

AGE IS AN ATTITUDE OF MIND

General Douglas MacArthur, head of American forces in the Pacific in World War II, popularized Samuel Ullman's essay on youth, which embodies the qualities you should emulate on your journey towards ageing youthfully.

'Youth is not a period of life, but an attitude of mind. We do not grow old because we have lived for a certain number of years. We grow old if we give up our ideals.

'He is young who can still be astonished and enthusiastic, and who challenges events and rejoices in the game of life. You are as young as your faith, as old as your doubt. As young as your self-confidence. As young as your hope. As old as your depression.

'You will stay young as long as your readiness to take up a challenge remains; receptive to the beautiful, the good and the great; receptive to the message of nature, of your fellow man, of the mysterious.

'Should your heart one day become corroded by pessimism or cynicism, then may God have mercy on your soul – the soul of an old man.'

ACTION PLAN

➤ Prepare yourself for the 'age of living' – do not think of retiring.

➤ Cultivate centenarian qualities from early midlife, so that they become a way of living.

➤ Remember that a dose of laughter is medication for the soul.

➤ Keep your life in balance. Daily self-examination will tell you which areas require attention.

➤ The alternative to premature ageing is to remain youthful at any age – the choice is entirely up to you.

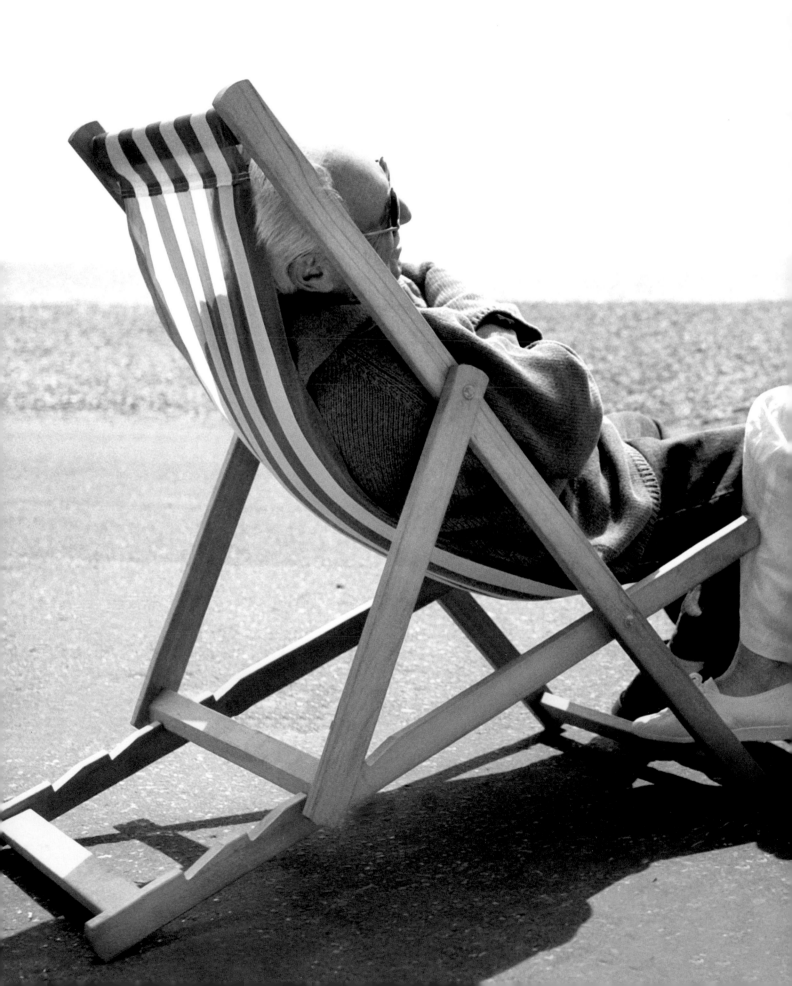

TODAY WELL LIVED MAKES EVERY TOMORROW A VISION
OF HOPE AND EVERY YESTERDAY A DREAM OF HAPPINESS.
(Sanskrit proverb)

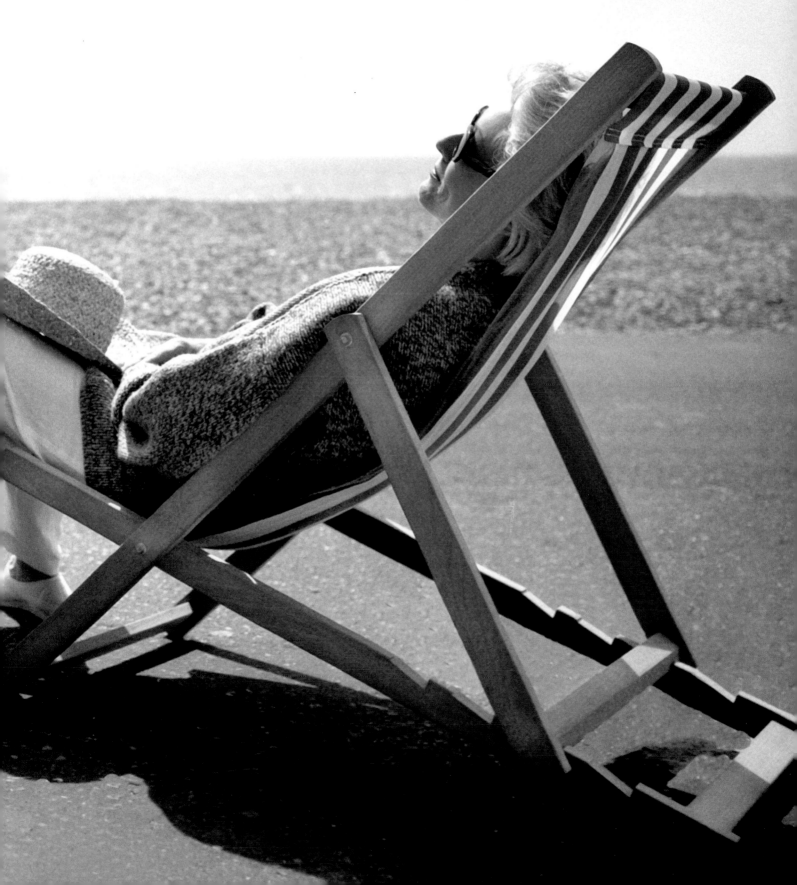

GLOSSARY

Adaptogen: a herbal supplement that helps adrenal glands cope with stress

Advanced glycosylated end products (AGEs): these occur when glucose combines with proteins in the blood and tissues, resulting in tissue damage – a process called glycosylation

Age-associated memory impairment (AAMI): form of memory loss often associated with ageing individuals and sometimes confused with early Alzheimer's disease

Andropause: male menopause, when a man's testosterone levels decrease after the age of 50

Antioxidants: found in fruit and vegetables, these compounds neutralize harmful effects of free radicals and protect against oxidative damage

Ayurveda: an Indian holistic medical system, also known as 'the science of life'

Biochemical individuality: each person's unique metabolism and nutritional needs

Biomarkers: tests that assess the biochemical and biological status of the body in relationship to ageing

Body mass index (BMI): weight divided by height squared; used to estimate whether someone is normal or overweight

Bone mineral density: a radiological test to assess bone health, useful for diagnosing and monitoring osteoporosis

Brain Gym: series of physical exercises to improve memory, learning and brain functioning

Carcinogen: cancer-promoting substance

Centenarian: person who has reached 100 years

Chromosome: a long molecule, containing a number of genes, in each cell of the body

Colonic irrigation: method of removing waste from the large colon using water and a hose; also known as colon hydrotherapy or colon cleansing

Cortisol: the stress hormone released by the adrenal gland

C-reactive protein (CRP): levels are estimated by a blood test to detect any inflammatory process

Detoxification: eliminating toxins and cleansing the liver and intestines by means of following a restricted diet

Dehydroepiandrosterone (DHEA): adrenal steroid hormone that counteracts the effects of cortisol, fighting stress and promoting wellbeing; levels decrease with age

Essential fatty acids (EFAs): these include the important omega-3 and omega-6 fatty acids, which cannot be manufactured by the body, and must be obtained in the diet or by supplementation

Excitotoxin: an artificial flavouring agent that has a harmful effect on the brain

Female androgen deficiency syndrome: a lack or deficiency of the male hormone testosterone in females, associated with low libido and with fatigue

Ferritin: a blood test to check ferritin levels; reflects iron storage in the body

Free radical: harmful, reactive compound formed in the body by oxidation; damages cells and tissues

Free radical assessment system (FRAS): a laboratory test to estimate levels of free radicals in blood and urine, and indicate free-radical damage in the body

Glycosylation: the combination of glucose with protein in cells and tissues, forming a sticky compound that accelerates ageing

Glycosylated haemoglobin (HbA1C): blood test reflecting average blood sugar levels over a period of weeks

Glycaemic index (GI): a table comparing the effects of different foods on blood sugar levels; high-GI foods result in higher blood sugar levels than low-GI foods

Growth hormone (HGH): produced by the pituitary gland in decreasing amounts with ageing; treatment by injection improves body composition with decreased fat levels and an increase in lean tissue

Hara hachi bu: Okinawan practice of eating until 80 per cent full to avoid overeating and obesity

Hoover syndrome: overeating

Homocysteine: an amino acid found in the blood; high levels are a risk factor for heart disease

Insulin resistance: also known as Syndrome X or metabolic syndrome; increased levels of blood glucose may become resistant to the action of insulin; associated with diabetes, high blood pressure, abdominal obesity and increased risk of heart disease

Insulin-like growth factor (IGF-1): growth hormone is transformed into IGF-1 in the liver; acts as a partner to growth hormone, with similar actions

Leaky gut syndrome: increased intestinal permeability allowing foreign food particles to be absorbed through the gut lining

Lipogram: blood test estimating levels of cholesterol and blood fats or triglycerides

Melatonin: hormone produced by the pineal gland in the brain during sleep and darkness; has antioxidant and immune-boosting properties but levels decline with ageing

Mind map: pictorial and diagrammatic method of creative thinking, note-taking and problem solving

Multihormone replacement: practice of prescribing a cocktail of several male or female hormones together with other hormones, such as thyroid, DHEA, melatonin and growth hormone

Natural killer (NK) cells: white blood cells produced in the thymus gland for protection against bacteria, viruses and foreign invaders

Pelvic ultrasound: use of ultrasound to assess ovaries, uterine size and endometrial (inner lining of the uterus) thickness

Perimenopause: period in a woman's life prior to menopause, usually at age 45 to 50; characterized by hormone imbalance

Phyto-oestrogens: plant oestrogens, found in soy, red clover, black cohosh and flaxseed, that block the effects of excess oestrogen; used as an alternative to hormone replacement therapy

Pregnenalone: anti-stress hormone derived from cholesterol and a precursor of DHEA; levels decline with ageing; supplementation can improve memory

Prebiotic: food substances, such as fructo-oligosaccharides, which enhance the action of probiotics

Probiotics: food ingredients, such as lactobacilli in yoghurt, which encourage a healthy gut

Prostate specific antigen (PSA): a blood test for men to estimate prostate health and detect possible early prostate cancer

Psyllium: plant fibre that swells in contact with water, adding bulk to the diet and preventing constipation

Qi (or Chi): the Chinese word for energy, which flows through a series of channels or meridians in the body

Secretagogue: amino acids such as arginine and ornithine stimulate the pituitary gland to release growth hormone; used as oral supplements as an alternative to growth hormone injections

Synchronicity: meaningful coincidence

Telomere: found on the end of each chromosome; shortening of the telomeres accelerates cellular ageing

Telomerase therapy: treatment with the enzyme telomerase lengthens telomeres in order to prevent ageing and increase lifespan

Thalassotherapy: treatment with seawater and seaweed

Yin and yang: the law of opposites; Chinese traditional medicine aims to keep yin and yang in balance for optimum health and wellbeing

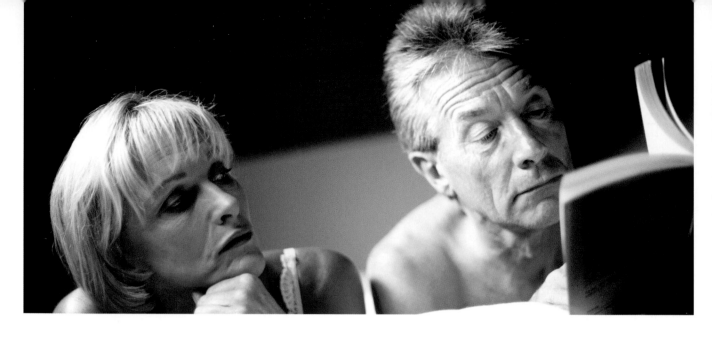

RECOMMENDED READING

Anderson, B. (2000). *Stretching*. Bolinos, California: Shelter Publications.

Brand-Miller, J. (1996). *The G.I. Factor*. Rydalmere, Australia: Hodder and Stoughton.

Buzan, T. (1983). *Use Both Sides of your Brain*. New York: E. P Dutton.

Cabot, S. (2000). *Menopause – Hormone Replacement Therapy and Natural Alternatives*. Cobbitty, Australia: Women's Health Advisory Service.

Cabot, S. (2001). *You Could Have Syndrome X*. Cobbitty, Australia: Women's Health Advisory Service.

Carper, J. (2000). *Your Miracle Brain*. London: Thorsons.

Carruthers, M. (1996). *Male Menopause*. London: Harper Collins.

Chopra, D. (2000). *Grow Younger Live Longer – 10 Steps to Reverse Ageing*. London: Ebury Press.

Crook, T. (1999). *The Memory Cure*. London: Thorsons.

De Jager, M. (2001). *Brain Gym for All*. Cape Town: Human and Rousseau.

Fossel, M. (1996). *Reversing Human Ageing*. New York: William Morrow & Co.

Haas, E. (1996). *The Detox Diet*. Berkley, California: Celestial Arts.

Hertoghe, T. (2002). *The Hormone Solution*. New York: Harmony Books.

Kelder, P. (1999). *Ancient Secret of the Fountain of Youth*. New York: Doubleday.

Khalsa, D.S. (1997). *Brain Longevity*. New York: Warner Books.

Kilham, C. (1994). *The Five Tibetans*. Rochester, USA: Healing Arts Press.

Klatz, R. (1999). *Ten Weeks to a Younger You*. Chicago: Sports Tech Labs Inc.

Klatz, R. (1999). *Hormones of Youth*. Chicago: Sports Tech Labs Inc.

Mahoney, D. and Restak, R. (1998). *The Longevity Strategy: Using the Brain-Body Connection*. New York: Wiley.

Moir, A. and Jessel, D. (1991). *Brain Sex*. New York: Dell Publishing.

Northrup, C. (1995). *Women's Bodies, Women's Wisdom*. London: Piatkus.

Pizzorno, J. (1998). *Total Wellness*. Rocklin, USA: Prima Publishing.

Rueff, D. (1998). *La Bible Anti-Age* (in French). Geneva: Editions Jouvence.

Sapolsky, R. (1998). *Why Zebras don't get Ulcers*. New York: W.H. Freeman.

Sears, B. (1999). *The Anti-Ageing Zone*. London: Harper Collins.

Serfontein, W. (2001). *New Nutrition*. Cape Town: Tafelberg.

Willcox, B. and Suzuki, M. (2000). *The Okinawa Way*. London: Penguin / Michael Joseph.

Yanick, P. and Giampapa, V. (1997). *Quantum Longevity*. San Diego: Promotion Publishing.

WEBSITES

ANTI-AGEING ORGANIZATIONS
American Academy of Anti-Ageing Medicine:
    www.worldhealth.net
European Academy of Quality of Life and
    Longevity Medicine: www.eaquall.net

AGEING AND HEALTH
British Geriatric Society: www.bgs.org.uk
National Institute on Ageing (USA):
    www.nih.gov/nia
Mayo Clinic (USA): www.mayohealth.org
British Longevity Society:
    www.antiageing.freeserve.co.uk
Foundation for Integrated Medicine (UK):
    www.fimed.org
Foundation for Integrated Medicine (USA):
    www.mdheal.org

CENTENARIAN STUDIES
New England Centenarian Study:
    www.med.harvard.edu/programs/necs
Okinawa Centenarian Study: www.okicent.org

DEMENTIA
National Parkinson's Foundation (USA):
    www.parkinson.org
Alzheimer's Association (USA): www.alz.org
Alzheimer's Society (UK): www.alzheimers.org.uk
Alzheimer's Australia NSW: www.alznsw.asn.au

MENOPAUSE AND ANDROPAUSE
Women's Health Advisory Service (Australia):
    www.whas.com.au
Andropause Society (UK): www.andropause.org.uk
Androscreen Information Center (USA):
    www.androscreen.com

SPECIALIZED LABORATORY TESTS
Great Smokies Laboratory (USA): www.gsdl.com
Biolab Medical Unit (UK): www.biolab.co.uk

OSTEOPOROSIS AND ARTHRITIS
National Osteoporosis Society (UK):
    www.nos.org.uk
National Osteoporosis Foundation (USA):
    www.nof.org
Arthritis Foundation (USA): www.arthritis.org

SPAS
World spas (USA): www.worldspas.com
Spas only (USA): www.spasonly.com
Spa-quest (USA): www.spa-quest.com
British spas (UK): www.spafinders.co.uk

HERBAL REMEDIES AND SUPPLEMENT SUPPLIER
The Nutricentre (UK): www.nutricentre.co.uk

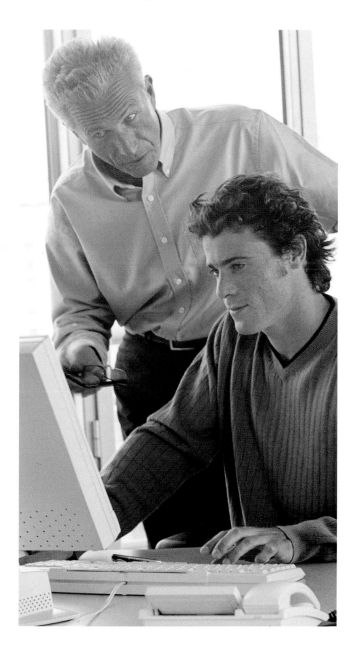

INDEX

Illustrations appear in bold